OXFORD MEDICAL PUBLICATIONS

**Geriatric problems
in general practice**

OXFORD GENERAL PRACTICE SERIES

Editorial board

G. H. FOWLER, J. A. M. GRAY,
J. C. HASLER, J. P. HORDER,
D. C. MORRELL

1. Paediatric problems in general practice
   M. Modell and R. D. H. Boyd
2. Geriatric problems in general practice
   G. K. Wilcock, J. A. M. Gray, and P. M. M. Pritchard
3. Prevention in general practice
   edited by J. A. M. Gray and G. H. Fowler
4. Women's problems in general practice
   edited by A. McPherson and A. Anderson

In preparation
   Locomotor disorders in general practice
   edited by M. I. V. Jayson and R. Million
   The consultation: an approach to learning and teaching
   D. Pendleton, P. H. L. Tate, P. B. Havelock, and T. P. C. Schofield
   The health care of immigrants
   edited by C. Ferreyra and B. Jarman
   The management of chronic disease
   edited by J. C. Hasler and T. P. C. Schofield
   Management in general practice
   P. M. M. Pritchard, K. Low, and M. Whalen

Geriatric problems in general practice

Oxford General Practice Series 2

G. K. WILCOCK
*Consultant Physician,
Radcliffe Infirmary,
Oxford, and Clinical Lecturer in
General and Geriatric Medicine,
University of Oxford*

J. A. M. GRAY
*Community Physician,
Oxfordshire Area Health Authority*

P. M. M. PRITCHARD
*General Practitioner,
Oxfordshire*

OXFORD
OXFORD UNIVERSITY PRESS
NEW YORK   TORONTO   MELBOURNE
1982

Oxford University Press, Walton Street, Oxford OX2 6DP

London Glasgow New York Toronto
Delhi Bombay Calcutta Madras Karachi
Kuala Lumpur Singapore Hong Kong Tokyo
Nairobi Dar es Salaam Cape Town
Melbourne Auckland

and associate companies in
Beirut Berlin Ibadan Mexico City Nicosia

© G. K. Wilcock, J. A. M. Gray, and P. M. M. Pritchard, 1982

All rights reserved. No part of this publication may be reproduced, stored in a retrieval system, or transmitted, in any form or by any means, electronic, mechanical, photocopying, recording, or otherwise, without the prior permission of Oxford University Press.

British Library Cataloguing in Publication Data

Wilcock, G.K.
  Geriatric problems in general practice.
  —(Oxford medical publications).—(Oxford general practice series; 2)
  1. Geriatrics
  I. Title   II. Gray, J.A.M.
  III. Pritchard, P.M.M.
  618.97   RC952

ISBN 0-19-261313-8

Library of Congress Cataloguing in Publication Data

Wilcock, G.K. (Gordon, K.)
  Geriatric problems in general practice.
  (Oxford general practice series; 2) (Oxford medical publications)
  Bibliography: p.
  Includes index.
  1. Geriatrics. I. Gray, J. A. Muir (John Armstrong Muir).
II. Pritchard, P. M . M. (Peter M. M.)
III. Title. IV. Series: Oxford general practice series; no. 2.
V. Series: Oxford medical publications.
[DNLM: 1. Family practice. 2. Geriatrics. W1 OX55 no. 2/WT 100 W667ga]
RC952.W45   618.97   82-6445

ISBN 0-19-261313-8 (pbk.)   AACR2

Photoset by Cotswold Typesetting Ltd., Cheltenham
Printed in Hong Kong

Preface

Most people who work with older patients are caught in a paradox. On the one hand they argue that older people are not qualitatively different from younger people and require a similar approach: the same quality of service, the same respect, the same honesty, and same standard of clinical practice. On the other hand they argue that people *are* significantly different and that their needs are such that they should be given priority for resources, and that doctors and other professionals require special training for their care. In part this paradox can be explained by the fact that most of those who are particularly interested in the problems of older people feel that it is necessary to emphasize that older people are the same, because so many of those who do not have a special interest appear to assume that they are different from younger people by being unable to change or learn, that they are beyond rehabilitation, 'dementing' and 'senile'. Similarly there is a need to argue the case for more services for older people simply to bring them up to the quality of services for other patient groups.

These points only partly explain the paradox. The principal explanation is that the paradox does not really exist at all. Elderly people are the same as younger people; it is elderly *patients* that are different from younger patients. The signs and symptoms of disease, the physical response to disease or trauma or treatment, and the beliefs and attitudes of older patients are slightly, but significantly, different and it is these differences we have tried to summarize in this book.

Furthermore, we have tried to write the book for the doctor seeing, treating, and supporting the elderly person in his own home and that doctor is, of course, the general practitioner. Without junior medical colleagues, pressed for time, without easy access to investigative services, often without the opportunity to undress the patient in warmth and comfort and assailed by the social problems that so often complicate disease in old age the general practitioner has to make the critical decisions. We hope this book will help him to do so.

Our special thanks are due to our families for their support while this book was in preparation, and to Rosemary Lees for her help in producing the book.

Oxford   G.K.W.
June 1982   J.A.M.G.
  P.M.M.P.

Contents

1. Introduction — 1
2. The aging process — 14
3. Management of common problems in the elderly — 18
4. Prescribing for the elderly — 90
5. The pattern of services — 100
6. Are older patients different? — 112
7. Prevention in old age — 127
8. Family problems — 138
9. Common handicaps — 156
10. Social problems — 171
11. Practical issues facing the general practitioner in caring for the elderly — 199
    Peter Pritchard
12. Terminal care in the home — 219
    Roy Spilling

Appendix 1. Useful addresses — 233
Appendix 2. The coroner — 236
Appendix 3. Compulsory institutionalization — 237
Appendix 4. A table of normal values in the elderly — 239
References — 241
Index — 245

1 Introduction

THE CHALLENGE FOR GENERAL PRACTICE

> The role of the family doctor is therefore of crucial and increasing importance if more elderly people are to be enabled to live independent lives in their own homes (or with some support from their families) (DHSS 1981).

'By the end of the century the number of people aged 75 and over is expected to increase by about one-fifth and the number aged 85 and over by no less than one half.' This simple sentence in the second paragraph of the Government's 1981 White Paper 'Growing Older' (Department of Health 1981) emphasizes the size of the challenge which is facing members of the medical profession and society as a whole (Arie 1981).

The medical implications of this demographic change are certainly daunting, as health service statistics illustrate. For example, the utilization of hospital bed days increases dramatically with age, with the shape of the graph being almost exponential (Fig. 1.1). The change in the age-specific incidence rates for

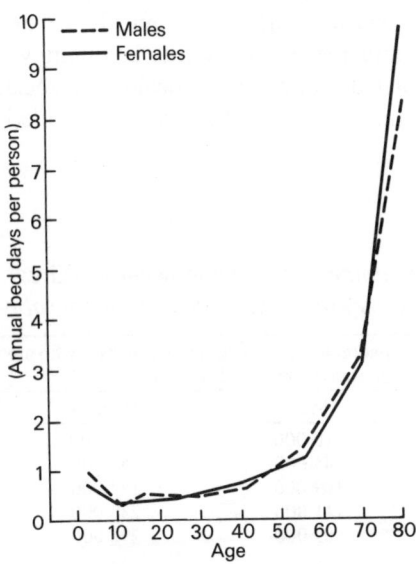

Fig. 1.1. Use of hospital beds (excluding maternity) by patients in different age groups. (From *Population trends* No. 3. HMSO, London (1976).)

2 Introduction

Table 1.1. *Average annual rate of fracture Dundee and Oxford combined 1954–8*

Age group	Upper end of humerus Male	Upper end of humerus Female	Neck of femur Male	Neck of femur Female
35–44	1.5	0.6	−z	0.2
45–54	2.7	2.1	0.5	0.7
55–64	3.3	5.5	1.6	1.5
65–74	4.3	8.3	2.7	7.4
75–84	8.7	21.3	7.4	24.1
85+	28.8	30.1	17.3	66.2

From Knowleden, J., Buhn, A. J., and Dunbar, O. (1964). Incidence of fractures in persons over 35 years of age – a report to the MRC working party on fractures in the elderly. *Br. J. Prev. Soc. Med.* **18**, 130–41.

fractures, to take a common reason for hospital attendance and admission, shows this trend clearly (Table 1.1).

In the psychiatric hospitals the impact of age is even more marked; a quarter of the beds are now occupied by patients aged over 75 (Department of Health 1981). The prevalence of chronic disabling disease shows the same pattern: two-thirds of all severely or appreciably handicapped people are over the age of 65, and of the very severely handicapped two-thirds are over 75 (Table 1.2) (Harris 1971).

The population is aging and the demand for hospital services will increase. However, it seems very unlikely that any developed country will be able to expand its hospital services sufficiently quickly to keep pace with these demographic trends and the trend towards community care will necessarily increase making greater demands on the health and social services, voluntary services, and, most important of all, the relatives of elderly people and elderly people themselves.

Table 1.2. *Estimated numbers of men and women in Great Britain of different ages who are very severely, severely or appreciably handicapped*

Age group	Men	Women	Men and women
16–29	10 000	9000	19 000
30–49	45 000	52 000	97 000
50–64	109 000	172 000	281 000
65–74	111 000	238 000	349 000
75 and over	89 000	292 000	381 000
All age groups*	365 000	763 000	1 128 000

*Totals may differ from sum of columns due to rounding
From Harris, A. (1971). *Handicapped and impaired in Great Britain*, p. 14. HMSO, London.

THE NATURE OF THE PROBLEM

We have used the word 'challenge' rather than some of the more pessimistic terms which have been used to describe the impact of this aging of the population because we believe that many people have been too pessimistic and that although there is no doubt that the numbers of aged people are going to increase dramatically that does not mean that the numbers of disabled elderly people will increase at the same rate.

There are two principal reasons why the future should not be so difficult as many people think. The first is that the old people of the future, namely ourselves, will not be the same as the old people of today. Their physical condition and mental outlook on life will be different. The elderly people of today are a cohort in which physical disease has been common at all ages and many suffered from rheumatic fever, bronchiectasis, often as a complication of measles, mastoiditis, and malnutrition, to list only a few of the conditions which are now much less common. The cohort which is becoming old, although it is affected by 'newer' diseases, notably those caused by cigarette smoking, should be much fitter in old age. In addition, the beliefs and attitudes of those who are growing old are different from those who are old today and this is of particular importance to the general practitioner (see p. 112).

The second reason why we are optimistic is that we believe that the amount which can be done to prevent and treat disease and disability has been underestimated. Aging is a normal, biological process which cannot be prevented or treated, but three other processes which cause disability and handicap can be treated – disease, unfitness, and the social consequences of growing old in our society (Fig. 1.2).

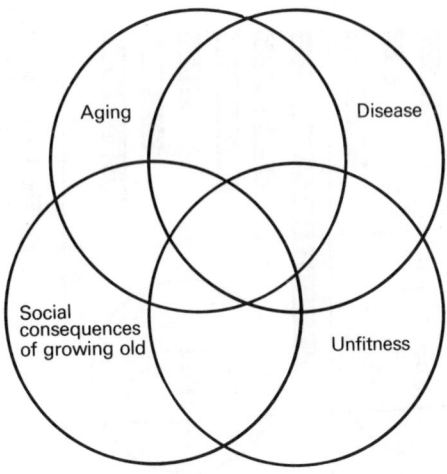

Fig. 1.2. The four processes of old age.

4 Introduction

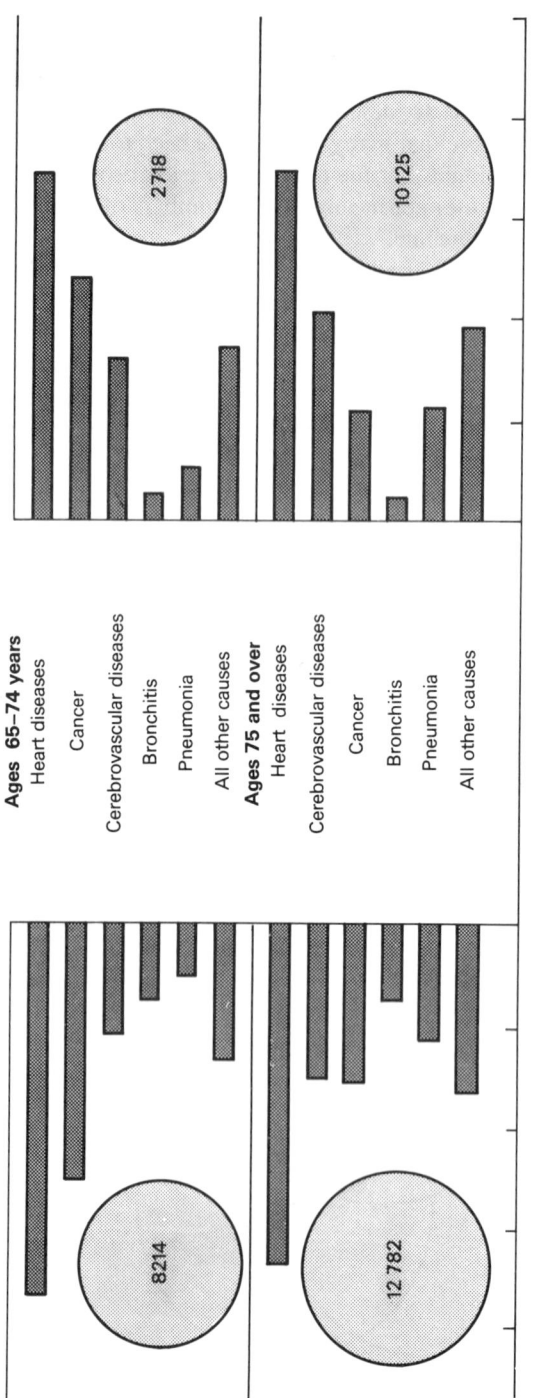

Fig. 1.3. Causes of death in old age. Figures in circles represent the death rates from *all causes* in 1973 per 100 000 population in each age and sex group. (From *Social trends*. HMSO, London (1975).).

Aims and objectives of medicine in old age

In this book we have tried to summarize what can be done to prevent and treat disease, unfitness, and the social consequences of growing old.

AIMS AND OBJECTIVES OF MEDICINE IN OLD AGE

The common causes of death in old age are shown in Fig. 1.3, although the notorious unreliability of death certificates for old people must be borne in mind when considering these data.

However, the prolongation of life is not one of the principal objectives of medicine in old age; as the motto of the British Geriatrics Society pithily states the objective is usually to 'Add life to years, not years to life'. Some old people are afraid of death but many are not so much frightened by death as by the prospect of disability, of becoming 'a burden' or 'a cabbage'. Indeed some old people look forward to death with pleasure, either because it will relieve them from their present suffering – 'I often wish I could just not wake up' – or because they are looking forward to meeting a dead spouse, brothers, or sisters in the life after death.

In spite of the fact that there has been criticism of the medical profession for 'keeping old people alive too long' there is little evidence that this takes place to any significant degree. The expectation of life of old people has not increased dramatically since the introduction of the National Health Service and it is important to appreciate that there was an increase in the expectation of life before 1948 (Fig. 1.4).

The increase, although small, has been significant for general practitioners because of the high incidence and prevalence of disabling disease. However, the increase in the number of elderly people need not be accompanied by an increase in the numbers of disabled people, because much of disability is caused

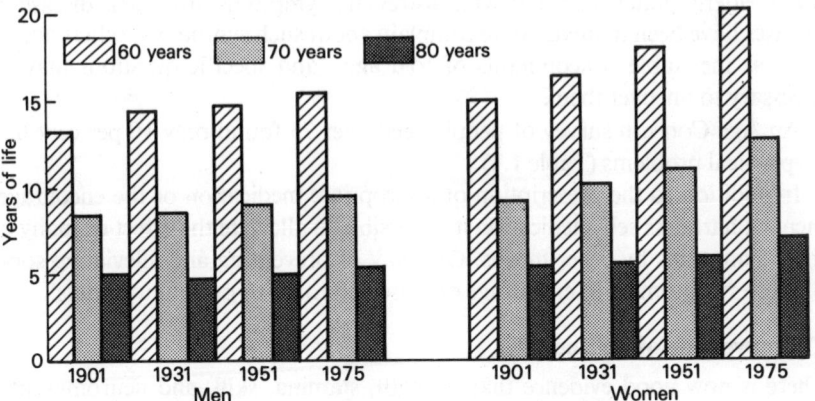

Fig. 1.4. Expectancy of life in Great Britain.

by disease and unfitness and one authority has pointed out that even though medicine cannot influence the age of mortality significantly it can postpone the age of onset of disability so that the period of terminal dependency is decreased in length with a fit old age being followed by a short period of dependency before death. The aim of medicine is therefore to improve the quality of life of older people.

The importance of good health to old people is difficult to overestimate and one sound study of the sources of satisfaction in old age, and the degree to which they were attained, showed clearly how important good health is – second only to 'good neighbours and friends' – and how seldom it is attained (Table 1.3).

In the words of the author of this report, Mark Abrams, 'Clearly, medical care has a very long part to play in determining the quality of life of old people' and he emphasized that health, although second in the list of sources of satisfaction, was lowest in the list when the degree of attainment was assessed.

The main aim of medicine is therefore to improve the quality of life and this aim can be broken down into a number of specific objectives:

More effective control of disease.
More effective symptom control.
The prevention of unfitness.
The prevention of dependence and handicap.

More effective control of disease

This is obviously the foundation of clinical work with older people and is the main theme of this book. However, many diseases are incurable and attention must therefore be paid to the sequelae of disease – symptoms, unfitness, and disability.

More effective symptom control

Many elderly patients are left with distressing symptoms after their disease or diseases have been treated. Some complain about such symptoms, others accept them as inevitable concomitants of 'old age', and specific questions may be necessary to uncover them.

An Age Concern survey of people aged over 75 found only 10 per cent had no physical problems (Table 1.4).

In addition to the prescription of appropriate medication or the encouragement of harmless self-medication it is possible to alleviate the effect of many of these symptoms by other means. One way of preventing and alleviating some of these symptoms is to encourage exercise and to try to prevent unfitness.

The prevention of unfitness

There is now good evidence that strength, stamina, skill, and neuromuscular co-ordination can be improved in older people by a programme of fitness training (p. 130). Furthermore, old people who participate in such programmes

Aims and objectives of medicine in old age 7

Table 1.3. *How far satisfaction criteria attained:* all aged 65 or more*

Potential source of real satisfaction	Proportion naming each source (%)	Degree of attainment				N
		Great extent (%)	Certain extent (%)	Hardly at all (%)	Not at all (%)	
Happy marriage, family	14.1	77	17	2	4 =100%	232
Helping others	3.7	70	25	4	1	60
Content with lot	11.3	68	28	2	2	186
Sun, warm weather	0.5	67	33	–	–	8
Miscellaneous reason	16.8	66	24	6	4	277
Peace, quiet, solitude	3.8	55	37	4	4	63
Good neighbours and freinds	18.4	51	34	12	3	303
Able to get out and about	5.4	48	30	16	6	89
Enough money	9.2	44	37	12	7	151
Good health	14.7	39	46	12	3	242
Total †	97.9	Weighted average 58	30	8	4	1611

*In order to obtain a numerically adequate base for each named source of satisfaction this table relates to *all* respondents in the survey.

† Total excludes those who said either that nothing could make for satisfaction in old age, or that they were unable to think of any possible source.

From Abrams, M. (1978). *Beyond three score and ten,* p. 53. Age Concern.

Table 1.4. *Proportions suffering from various ailments among people aged 75 or more: England 1977*

(expressed as a percentage)

Arthritis, rheumatism	58
Unsteady on feet	49
Forgetfulness	44
Poor eyesight	42
Hard of hearing	36
Backache	36
Breathless after any effort	35
Swelling of feet, legs	33
Giddiness	31
Indegestion, flatulence	29
Always feel tired	29
Heart trouble	21
High blood pressure	21
Headaches	20
Constipation	19
Breathless at night	19
Stomach trouble	18
Long spells depression	14
Incontinence	11
Toothache, gum trouble	6
Difficulty passing water	5
No. of ailments, average responce	5.8
No physical problems	10

From Abrams, M. (1978). *Beyond three score and ten,* p. 55. Age Concern.

8   Introduction

report an improvement in morale and feelings of wellbeing and these psychological effects may be equally important in the prevention of symptoms such as tiredness and backache.

People who develop a disabling disease are more likely to become unfit than those who do not suffer from chronic disease. There are too few physiotherapists working outside hospital to give such people the type of help they need and it is often left to the general practitioner to offer advice and encouragement to the disabled old person who would benefit if her fitness were improved.

Prevention of disability and handicap (see p. 156)

These terms are often used as though they were synonymous but it has now been agreed internationally that they should be used to denote different conditions and this distinction is useful in practice. A *disability* is any restriction or lack of ability to perform an activity in the manner or within the range considered normal for someone of that person's age. For example, the limited hip flexion resulting from osteoarthritis or the limitation in movement and power of the upper limb resulting from the spasticity and contractures on the side of the body affected by a cerebrovascular accident (Wood 1980).

A *handicap* is a disadvantage, such as difficulty with dressing, or preparing food, or reaching the toilet unaided, resulting from a disability. Whether or not a disabled person will be handicapped as a result of her disability is determined not only by the degree of her disability. It is also influenced by her physical environment and by social factors. A person who is so disabled by osteoarthritis of the hips that she cannot climb stairs will be handicapped if she lives in a dwelling in which it is necessary to climb stairs to reach the toilet and bathroom. If that person is rehoused in a dwelling which has no stairs her handicap will be cured even though there has been no change in her degree of disability. The extent to which an individual will be handicapped by her disability is also influenced by the manner in which she has adapted to her disability and by her relationships with other people. With the same degree of disability some people are very much more handicapped than others.

A third term is of particular importance – *dependence*. A disabled elderly person who lives with relatives, or who has nearby relatives or neighbours who are willing to help her by performing the tasks which she cannot do may not be handicapped, but she will be dependent. Dependence can create problems both for the elderly person and for those on whom she has become dependent.

This distinction between disability and handicap is useful because it allows the contributions of the doctor, physiotherapist, and occupational therapist to be planned in logical sequence. The task of the general practitioner who is faced with a person who is handicapped is to try to minimize the disability by accurate diagnosis, appropriate treatment, and by ensuring that the person complies with treatment. To do this he may have to refer the person to hospital particularly if he is unable to request physiotherapy without hospital assessment. Once doctor and physiotherapist have done as much as they can to reduce the impairment resulting from the disabling disease the occupational therapist can then make her contribution. The objective of occupational therapy is to prevent and cure handicap by helping the disabled person adapt to her environment.

There are two common handicaps in old age – mobility problems and difficulties with self-care.

Mobility problems

Loss of mobility is a central problem in old age which gives rise to many other problems. Mobility problems are more common in women and obviously increase with age (Fig. 1.5).

Audrey Hunt who conducted the survey quoted emphasized the importance of immobility by saying that 'one-quarter of those unable to go out, even with assistance, live on their own and are therefore dependent on outsiders for everything that needs to be obtained away from their homes' (Hunt 1978). Furthermore, 42.5 per cent of the bedfast and housebound had not been out of the house for over a year and 18.9 per cent had not been out for over three years.

The causes of these mobility problems were also determined by the survey and what it clearly revealed was that very few people withdraw or 'disengage'

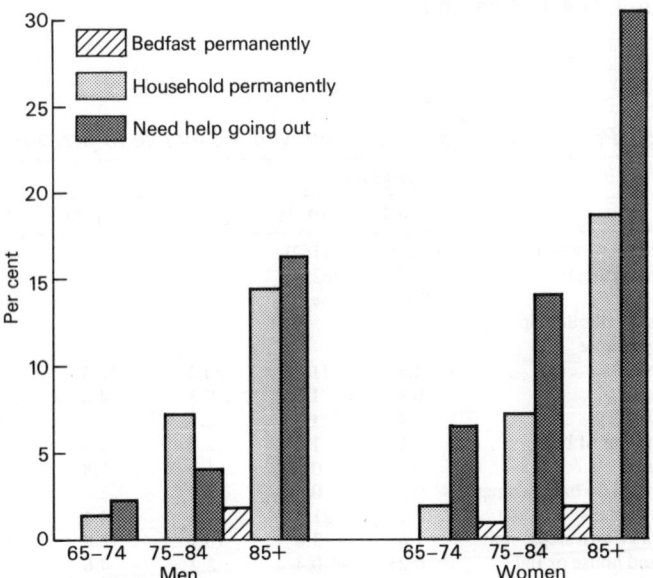

Fig. 1.5. Percentage of men and of women with loss of mobility in each age group. (From Hunt, A. (1978). *The elderly at home,* p. 69. HMSO, London.)

10 Introduction

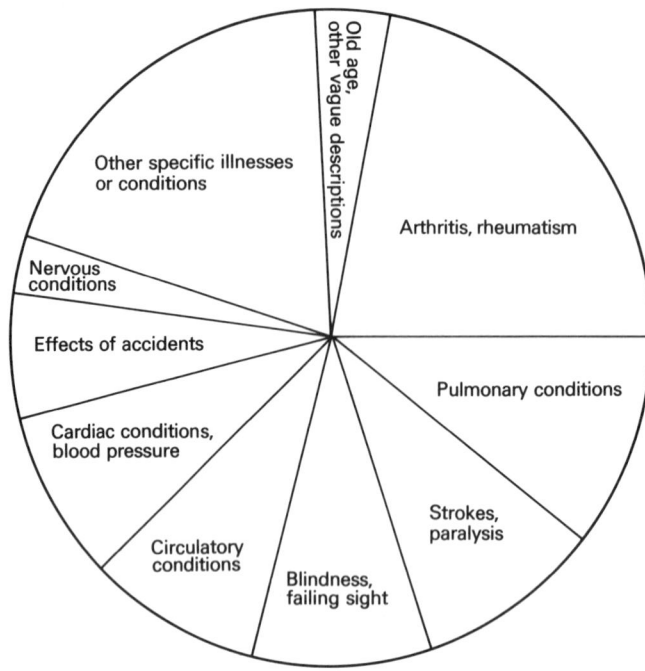

Fig. 1.6. Causes of being bedfast or housebound. (From Hunt, A. (1978). *The elderly at home*, p. 7. HMSO, London.)

Table 1.5. *Percentage in each age-group who are unable to perform each task*

	Age-group				
	65–69	70–74	75–79	80–84	85 and over
Elderly persons WEIGHTED	(1409)	(1162)	(679)	(392)	(209)
(unweighted figures)	(725)	(629)	(688)	(375)	(205)
	(%)	(%)	(%)	(%)	(%)
Unable to do without help					
or to totally unable					
Bath oneself	4.4	11.7	20.2	32.6	51.2
Wash oneself	0.8	1.0	2.3	4.6	7.2
Get to lavatory	0.4	1.3	2.8	5.1	6.2
Get in and out of bed	0.6	1.1	2.7	4.4	4.8
Feed oneself	0.1	0.3	1.3	1.8	2.4
Shave (men), do hair (women)	0.5	0.6	2.5	3.8	4.3
Cut own toenails	12.5	21.3	34.6	42.4	56.9
Get up and down steps, stairs	1.6	3.8	10.1	12.8	18.6
Get around house or flat	0.2	0.8	2.2	4.6	6.2
Go out of doors on own	4.4	9.5	16.5	23.5	48.9
Use public transport	5.3	9.3	15.1	23.8	37.9

From Hunt, A. (1978). *The elderly at home*, p. 74. HMSO, London.

Aims and objectives of medicine in old age 11

from society voluntarily as certain sociologists once argued. Most are immobilized by medical problems (Fig. 1.6).

Self-care problems

The survey revealed that the most difficult self-care tasks were cutting toenails and bathing (Table 1.5). In addition the research workers asked about the ability to perform domestic tasks and showed the difficulties which old people have with house repairs and maintenance, for which there is of course no statutory help (Table 1.6).

Table 1.6. *Percentages unable to perform each task (by sex and age, housewives and those living alone shown separately)*

	Total	Age				
		65–69	70–74	75–79	80–84	85 and over
Elderly persons WEIGHTED	(3869)	(1409)	(1162)	(697)	(392)	(209)
(unweighted figures)	(2622)	(725)	(629)	(688)	(375)	(205)
	(%)	(%)	(%)	(%)	(%)	(%)
Unable to						
Open screw-top bottles*	9.7	5.3	8.4	11.5	18.4	24.4
Do little sewing jobs*	14.9	9.7	11.8	17.1	27.6	35.4
Jobs involving climbing	43.0	28.0	37.7	57.1	67.3	80.4
Use a frying pan	5.4	2.1	2.8	6.0	13.8	24.9
Make a cup of tea	2.6	0.9	1.4	2.9	6.4	12.9
Cook a main meal	8.8	4.6	6.8	10.0	18.1	26.8
Cut the lawn †	25.8	15.7	20.9	33.4	47.2	56.0
Do heavy jobs in garden †	47.1	38.4	44.5	55.2	61.0	67.9
Do light jobs in garden †	19.3	10.0	15.4	27.0	34.7	49.8
Sweep floors	11.3	5.5	8.0	14.8	23.2	34.4
Wash floors	21.7	10.9	15.0	30.8	42.6	62.2
Make fires, carry fuel †	6.0	3.1	4.3	8.6	11.2	17.2
Wash clothes	14.5	6.8	10.8	20.2	29.1	39.7
Clean windows inside	23.6	11.4	17.6	32.3	48.0	65.1
Clean windows outside †	52.5	37.2	50.4	64.0	76.3	84.7
Wash paintwork	23.9	11.6	16.3	32.3	50.5	70.8
Minor repairs (e.g. fuses)	49.8	35.3	46.0	62.0	73.2	84.2
Repairs and redecoration inside	60.5	11.4	58.3	77.6	87.5	94.3
Repairs and redecoration outside †	49.2	12.0	46.6	53.7	65.6	65.6

*Bedfast informants were asked about these tasks. They are assumed to be unable to do the others.

† Informants who would not have to perform these tasks (e.g. because they had no garden) are included in the base figures so that the figures given show the percentages of all elderly for whom the tasks present problems. The percentages to whom these do not apply are: lawn 29.7 per cent, garden 22.6 per cent, solid fuel fires 55.8 per cent, windows outside 3.1 per cent, redecorations outside 35.9 per cent.

From Hunt, A. (1978). *The elderly at home*, p. 81. HMSO, London.

NEED AND DEMAND

The demands made by old people on general practitioners are heavy but the increase in demand with age is smaller than would be expected when the increase in morbidity is considered (Fig. 1.7). Demand increases but not, it would appear, in proportion to need. Furthermore there is evidence that the demand is falling (Table 1.7).

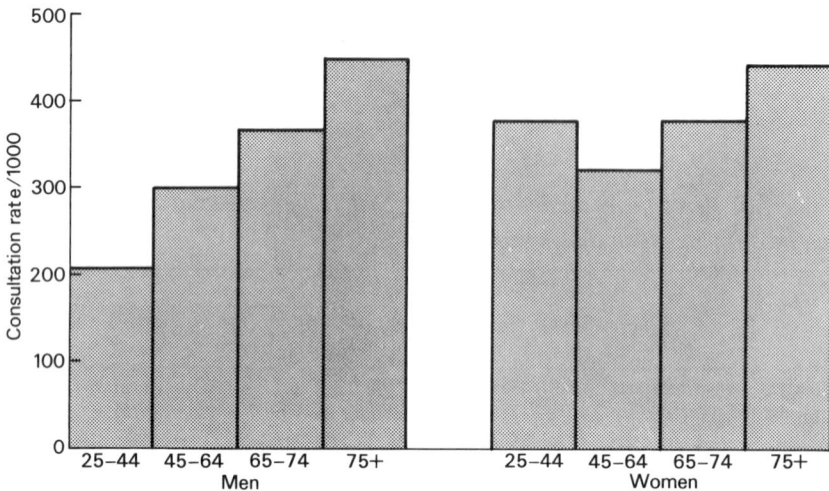

Fig. 1.7. Consultation rates per 1000 population. (From Morbidity statistics from general practice. Studies on medical and population studies No. 14. HMSO, London.)

Numerous surveys have shown the amount of unreported need among old people at home (Rowntree 1947; Sheldon 1948; Brockington and Lampert 1966). The survey of old people in Edinburgh reported by Professor Williamson and his colleagues was one of the first careful studies and it revealed that 'men had a mean of 3.26 disabilities of which 1.87 were unknown to the family doctors; women a mean of 3.42 disabilities with 2.03 unknown' (Williamson *et al.*, 1964).

Table 1.7. *Average percentage change in rate between 1971 and 1978 as percentage of 1971 rate—Great Britain*

Age group	Consultation	Attendances	Visits
45–64	−1.0	+8.6	−38.9
65–74	−17.5	−11.5	−28.5
75 and over	−29.3	−19.8	−34.9

Derived from the general household survey in Billsborough, J. S. (1981). Do patients consult the doctor less often than they used to? *J. R. Coll. Gen. Pract.* **31**, 91–105.

The reasons for the low level of demand among elderly people are complex. Some are due to trends in general practice which inhibit demand but the more important factors are the beliefs and attitudes of old people themselves. For this reason we need to consider the ways in which older patients differ from those of working age, physically, socially, and psychologically (see p. 112).

2 The aging process

Aging does not occur throughout all the species of the animal kingdom. There are many species of animal who never experience the phenomenon of normal senescence since natural forces intervene during their life-span and end their existence, not necessarily prematurely, but before the phenomenon of senescence can take hold. In the smaller species especially, a large percentage of animals never even reach maturity. Although the absence of a senescent phase in their life-history is more characteristic of smaller than larger animals, this is not always the case, e.g. many African elephants often die because their teeth wear out and they are unable to feed, rather than because of other diseases creeping up on them. Old age as a condition of mankind has probably arisen through the evolutionary processes. This is probably, at least in part, the result of fewer selection pressures against it, since human beings have learnt to control or avoid those factors which bring about earlier death.

CHRONOLOGICAL AND BIOLOGICAL AGE

Most people are aware that whilst certain individuals look their age others appear younger or older than their years. It is often possible to overestimate or underestimate a patient's age by as much as one or two decades. If the appearance is paralleled by similar changes in the body's physiological and anatomical processes it is apparent that there will be a discrepancy between the biological age and a person's chronological age. Biological age, however, is difficult to measure, although at the simplest level it may be based upon a person's appearance. More complex and sophisticated methods of assessing this have been developed, some of which take into account the number of symptoms and signs of age-related diseases, and other phenomena that an individual is experiencing. Difficult though it may be to measure, it is often a much sounder foundation upon which to base the approach to a patient's medical problems than considering his chronological age alone.

An example of this has been the practice to exclude people over the age of 70 years from coronary care units. Decisions made upon this basis may affect whether a patient lives or dies, since it implies that an individual's biological and chronological age are the same when this is so often manifestly not the case. A woman of 71 is often little different from when she was 69. The general practitioner is usually the only medically trained observer able to make a valid decision about someone's biological age, and this is extremely important when referring a patient to hospital, especially a geriatric patient. It is extremely easy for a hospital doctor to be misled by a patient's age, and to assume that the ill person he sees before him has little, if any, meaningful life in the community. A patient who is admitted with bronchopneumonia and dehydration may look moribund, and severely incapacitated, but the family doctor is in a position to decide whether it is appropriate to attempt to return him to his previous station in life.

LONGEVITY

Claims have been made for extreme longevity in particular groups of people from time to time. This has been as much as double the normal life-span that most of us would like to expect with values of 150 years or more. More usually, however, the age is quoted at the time of death as in the region of 110 to 120 years. It is true that in the western world in particular more and more people are living into the eight, ninth, and tenth decades, and although in 1951 it was estimated that were only about 750 people aged 100 or over in Great Britain, 20 years later the 1971 census revealed that this number had risen to 2430. While many of these extremely aged people are dependent upon others for their existence and many live in an institution, there are plenty of others who are fit able bodied members of society, who look after themselves. The majority of claims for *extreme* old age, however, are probably untrue. Many areas where great longevity has been reported do not have local birth records at all, and where birth certification has been adopted its introduction is often after the apparent birth-date of the person claiming to be very ancient. Parish records have often been resorted to in these circumstances, and in some instances have been found to be faked. There is another source of inaccuracy involving the habit of some communities to name the children after the family name so that, for instance, both father and son may be called Robert Smith. It has been shown in certain instances that the parent's birth-date has been adopted by the child who is claiming to have lived for so long. Without adequate birth and death certification, claims are difficult to substantiate or refute, and it may be that a few of the claims are correct. As far as the inhabitants of Great Britain are concerned, the oldest age obtained so far is 112 years.

One's life-span depends upon complex interactions of physiological, psychological, and social factors. It may be of interest that in an American study the following characteristics were observed in a group of people who had lived longer than their colleagues – high IQ, financial security, a stable marriage, good general health, and a fulfilling role in society. It can be seen that medical factors are not the only important ones.

THEORIES OF AGING

There are at present two major schools of thought concerning the nature of the aging process. One of these assumes that aging is a programmed, genetically controlled process, or series of processes, which will inevitably take place given sufficient time. The second concept is that senescence is the result of the accumulation of random damage at a cellular level leading to disruption and disorganization of tissues and organs. There is not any definite objective proof giving overwhelming credence to either of these views, and senescence may well turn out to be a multifactorial process.

Amongst the evidence cited in favour of a genetically programmed process is the propensity for the children of parents who have lived longer than average to themselves be more likely to have an above average life-span. Also, although sex-linked genes do not seem to be the reason, an individual's sex plays an important part since women tend to live longer than men. In addition it has been shown that monozygotic twins are closer in age when they die than are dizygotic individuals. Also in favour of a genetic component is the finding in at least one strain of mice of a single genetic locus which is associated with longevity, and which is thought possibly to act on secondary factors.

The concept of an accumulation of unprogrammed abnormalities within body cells has been explored in many different ways. An early hypothesis was that of the accumulation of abnormalities of protein synthesis, for instance, associated with errors of amino-acid incorporation. Although one abnormality of amino-acid incorporation in a protein may not really matter, the accumulation of more than this might have serious consequences, especially when enzymes are being synthesized. Much of the evidence surrounding this attractive hypothesis is, however, contradictory. At a slightly different level, somatic mutations occurring at mitosis itself have also been examined in relation to the possibility of causing senescence through organ dysfunction. This has been shown to be of little practical importance as artificial induction of such mutations shown by aberrations at mitosis seem to have little effect on the physiology of the cells subsequently, and upon their life-span. Self-destruction by low-grade autoimmune mechanisms, as distinct from specific so called autoimmune disorders like DLE, has also been considered as a contributory factor for the aging process, but there is as yet no definite proof that this makes a major contribution to senescence. The accumulation of fatty pigments, especially of the lipfuscin type, has been noted to increase as age progresses, particularly in the cells of such organs as the heart, brain, kidneys, and liver. It was thought that this build-up may interfere with the normal functions of the cells by affecting the biochemical reactions which take place within intracellular structures. However, the pigment accumulation is not always present to the same extent in the same organs in different individuals, and does not appear to consistently correlate with biological age.

The endocrine system plays an important role during development and maturation of many animals, including man. It is therefore considered to have a possible role in the aging process. If this was so it could be caused by an abnormality occuring at one or more different places in the 'endocrine reflexes'. There is some evidence that the secretion of posterior pituitary hormones may have a bearing on longevity, and also that the tissue binding of certain hormones alters with age. More extensive research is, however, necessary before the significance of these findings can be understood.

3 Management of common problems in the elderly*

ANAEMIA

Although most doctors will accept a lower haemoglobin in older people as being normal than they would do in younger patients, there is no logical reason for this to be the case. For practical purposes, however, it is often necessary to adopt a cut-off point below which further investigation is necessary, and an anaemia less than 12 g per 100 ml of blood should be considered further, as also should any consistent downward trend, even if the level is above 12. It is all too easy to dismiss a low haemoglobin as being an expected finding in an old person and denying them the opportunity of appropriate treatment to an underlying condition which might well improve the quality of their life. As is usually the case, the assessment of an anaemia is facilitated by subdividing the anaemias on the basis of the mean corpuscular volume into microcytic, macrocytic, and normocytic types.

Microcytic anaemia

This is the commonest anaemia of old age and is nearly always due to iron deficiency. It is best confirmed by checking the serum iron and total iron-binding capacity, but if these are found to be normal it is necessary to consider other possiblities, in particular a sideroblastic anaemia, or more rarely a thalassaemia, and in these circumstances hospital referral is necessary. When detecting an iron-deficiency anaemia the first step in an older person is to exclude dietary inadequacy. This may be indicated in the history, or there may be other biochemical evidence of malnutrition. Gastric irritation and consequent blood loss is another frequent finding, especially when a patient is taking certain drugs, such as aspirin and the non-steroidal anti-inflammatory analgesics, e.g. indomethazine, phenylbutazone, etc. Gastric neoplasms and peptic ulcers also frequently turn out to be the cause for this type of anaemia. GI tract blood loss may be confirmed by finding positive faecal occult blood, but this test can be misleading, and if a gastro-intestinal cause for the anaemia is suspected, barium studies and possibly endoscopy are indicated. Although a gastric neoplasm is unlikely to be surgically treated, other conditions such as peptic ulceration respond well to treatment. If it is not possible or appropriate to arrange these then it is reasonable to prescribe a course of iron and observe the

*The problems are listed in alphabetical order.

results. In the case of a suspected peptic ulcer a trial of appropriate therapy may well prove beneficial and can be monitored by periodical faecal occult blood determinations, as well as a blood count. Other causes of iron deficiency include blood loss from other sites, malabsorption, and haemolysis.

Macrocytic anaemia

Vitamin B_{12} and folate deficiency are the commonest cause of the macrocytic anaemia in elderly people. Folic acid deficiency may be associated with some drugs, e.g. phenytoin and co-trimoxazole. In theory, before attributing a macrocytic anaemia to a deficiency of one of these, it is necessary to confirm the presence of megaloblastic change in the bone marrow. This is so because there are other causes of macrocytosis, including liver disease, thyroid disease, vitamin C deficiency, and even a high reticulocyte level, since immature red blood cells are larger than the normal corpuscle. If, however, an estimation of the serum B_{12} or folate reveals one of these to be low, it is often reasonable to prescribe the appropriate replacement therapy and monitor the result. If it is decided that both B_{12} and folate should be given, the B_{12} should be started first and the loading dose given as well. The folic acid can be prescribed subsequently.

If there is B_{12} or folate deficiency it is necessary to consider the possibility of malnutrition due to an inadequate diet or malabsorption, and if appropriate investigate accordingly. Barium studies and endoscopy are occasionally necessary, especially if there is a history of gastro-intestinal symptoms since carcinoma of the stomach occurs more frequently in people with a history of pernicious anaemia, and also Crohn's disease of the terminal ileum or another lesion here may well be interfering with the absorption of B_{12}. Less commonly, a barium meal and follow-through will reveal small bowel diverticula, which may also be responsible for B_{12} deficiency. It is, however, not appropriate to subject an old person to a barium meal simply because they have B_{12} deficiency, unless there is an indication to do so.

When following up a patient in whom pernicious anaemia has been confirmed, it is important to remember that there is an increased incidence of other autoimmune diseases, especially thyroid disorders, Addison's disease due to adrenal atrophy, rheumatoid arthritis, and diabetes mellitus.

Normochromic/normocytic anaemia

A normochromic/normocytic anaemia is usually a concomitant of chronic disease, the aetiology of which is often very difficult to elucidate. It would not be practical here to list all the potential underlying conditions and the appropriate investigations required. Amongst the more important are chronic renal failure, chronic infection especially subacute bacterial endocarditis and tuberculosis, collagenoses, and malignancy. Occasionally, a normochromic normocytic picture is the result of a haemolytic process in which case there will usually be other confirmatory evidence, such as an elevation of the urinary urobilinogen level and a film suggestive of haemolysis. There may also be signs of a reticulocyte response and an elevated serum bilirubin. Haemolysis is discussed further in the section on jaundice.

ARTHRITIC COMPLAINTS

The commonest causes of arthritis in the elderly are osteoarthrosis and rheumatoid arthritis, and in the case of the latter there is often a superimposed element of osteoarthrosis. Although touched on briefly elsewhere, each merits consideration in its own right.

Osteoarthrosis

The classical presentation of osteoarthrosis involves the complaints of pain, stiffness, and in some joints deformity. Inflammation in the usual sense is absent, but there may be an effusion and occasionally the joint may feel warm. In the latter case this is probably more frequently associated with local trauma than with the arthritis itself. Osteoarthrosis may also present in other ways, for instance as specific as the rupture of a Baker's cyst in the popliteal-fossa, producing a clinical picture simulating a DVT, or in the more general sense of impaired ability to perform the activities of daily life. It is unrealistic to expect to confirm the diagnosis radiologically in every diseased joint. However, an X-ray should be considered necessary whenever the symptoms are atypical, the possibility of pyogenic arthritis is considered, or where the expected response to therapy is not forthcoming.

Treatment

In the initial stages many geriatricians prescribe simple analgesics, such as Paracetamol, although this is considered inappropriate by some rheumatologists. Despite this many elderly patients appear to benefit from the pain relief that is gained, and are not exposed to the more hazardous side-effects of the non-steroidal anti-inflammatory drugs. If a trial of simple analgesics is unsatisfactory, non-steroidal anti-inflammatory preparations should be prescribed, but the side-effects, especially dyspepsia, gastrointestinal-tract bleeding, and fluid and salt retention must not be forgotten.

Physiotherapy is the other main-stay of treatment. This can be carried out in the patient's home in those areas where there is a domiciliary physiotherapy service, or otherwise in a physiotherapy department or a day hospital. This should not be considered just remedial, but also of preventive value. Physiotherapy can play a major contribution in preventing muscle weakness and wasting associated with arthritis.

More specific measures are sometimes necessary, depending upon the joints involved. In the case of the lower limb, dietary restriction in an obese patient may lead to significant weight loss and help relieve the symptoms of arthritis in the hip and the knee. Dietary measures unfortunately are often unsuccessful in the elderly. In the case of degenerative disease of the cervical spine a cervical collar is often beneficial, and it is not always appreciated that in many instances it should be worn at night as well as during the day. Similarly a lumbar corset may be necessary for degenerative changes in the lumber spine.

Sadly many elderly patients are denied consideration of surgical relief of their symptoms simply because they are regarded as too old by their medical attendants, or the orthopaedic surgeons involved. It is extremely important to remember that biological rather than chronological age is the relevant factor, and in any patient in whom medical treatment has failed to alleviate the symptoms surgical intervention should be considered. This is particularly important in arthritis of the lower limbs as loss of mobility may herald the end of independence for the patient concerned.

Rheumatoid arthritis

Rheumatoid arthritis infrequently arises for the first time in elderly patients, but it can often continue to flare-up in the later years, pursuing a course that began sometime in middle or earlier life. Most frequently, however, rheumatoid arthritis in the elderly is of the burned-out variety associated with superimposed osteoarthrosis. Should it start in old age the symptoms and joint disease can be quite severe, but in general there are fewer erosions and nodules than in younger patients. In addition the systemic manifestations are usually less predominant than in younger patients, although there will usually be a high ESR and a normochromic, normocytic anaemia.

Treatment

It is important to avoid prolonged bed-rest in older patients if this is at all possible, and especially necessary to remember the possibility of contracture development, which may require the use of a splint for an inflamed joint.

The non-steroidal anti-inflammatory preparations are usually the main-stay of treatment, but it is very necessary not to forget the side-effects mentioned earlier. If possible, phenylbutazone is best avoided because of the hazard of aplastic anaemia and bone-marrow depression. If steroids are used it is essential to reduce the dose as soon as possible to 7.5 mg of Prednisolone daily or less, in order to minimize the risk of steroid-induced side-effects.

Intra-articular injections must be performed with scrupulous attention to sterility as many elderly patients have an increased susceptibility to infection. Although it may be necessary to prescribe gold-therapy or penicillamine for rheumatoid arthritis in the elderly, these treatments are probably best reserved for hospital supervision, as the side-effects can be extremely toxic.

As in the case of osteoarthrosis, the physiotherapist plays an important part in treating patients with rheumatoid arthritis, but the occupational therapist is especially important in his or her role of helping the patient to overcome or come to terms with the difficulties experienced in activities of daily living.

When medical treatment is unsuccessful or a patient presents with a severely disorganized joint, an elderly patient should not be barred from consideration of a surgical procedure such as synovectomy or joint replacement.

Crystal synovitis

Gout and psuedogout are not infrequently encountered in the elderly. *Gout* is commoner in women, contrary to popular opinion, and it must not be forgotten that there may be an underlying blood dyscrasia as its cause. An elevated uric acid level alone does not confirm the diagnosis of gout, since this occurs commonly as manifestation of drug therapy, especially with thiazide diuretics. The diagnosis is usually confirmed by discovering the characteristic crystal deposits in an effusion from the joint.

As in younger patients, gout is treated with a non-steroidal anti-inflammatory agent initially, and occasionally colchicine. For longer-term maintainance treatment, Allopurinol is probably best, and in the first two or three months of prescription it is wise to give a prophylactic dose of a non-steroidal anti-inflammatory agent such as Indomethacin to counteract the acute attacks that may be precipitated.

The diagnosis of *psuedogout* is often made radiologically with the discovery of chondrocalcinosis on an X-ray of a joint, usually the knee. A definitive diagnosis, however, as in the case of gout, relies upon finding the appropriate crystals in an effusion from a joint. In this case pyrophosphate crystals are found. Pseudogout is usually in the elderly unassociated with other conditions, although both hyperparathyroidism and haemochromatosis may occur in association with it. These therefore should be considered and excluded in any patient in whom chondrocalcinosis has been found.

The treatment of acute attacks of discomfort in a patient with psuedogout is the same as in the case of a patient with gout. Often, however, aspiration of an effusion will abort the attack for reasons that are obscure.

BACKACHE

Confusion often exists about the causes of backache in the elderly since osteoporosis is a common finding and discomfort is commonly attributed to its presence. Osteoporosis on its own, however, probably rarely accounts for backache unless there is an accompanying crush fracture of one or more of the vertebrae. This cannot be satisfactorily diagnosed without an X-ray, even if there is typical girdle-like radiation of pain. It should be treated with analgesics, lumbar support, and physiotherapy. In the case of severe pain hospitalization or attendance at a Day Hospital may be necessary, but one should always remember that in the presence of a crush fracture other causes should be excluded, such as myeloma and secondary deposits. This is because the osteoporosis itself may not be responsible, since it is present in so many people without symptoms.

Other conditions which cause backache include osteoarthritis in the spine and the sacro-iliac joint. Many people, however, have signs consistent with the diagnosis of early spinal osteoarthritis without experiencing any symptoms and so one has to think carefully before attributing a person's discomfort to this cause. When it is responsible for back pain, there is often a history of trauma and it may be the latter rather than the arthritis itself that is symptomatic. In the case of the sacro-iliac joint the symptoms can often be relieved by local injection of local anaesthetic and/or hydrocortisone. Secondary deposits, especially from the lung, prostate, breast, and in myeloma, may cause back pain without vertebral collapse. It is important to look for the primary since in certain cases, e.g. breast and prostate, the patient may well be helped by hormone treatment. A useful pointer is that breast and prostatic deposits are often sclerotic, and in the case of prostatic carcinoma, a high alkaline and acid phosphatase indicates the probability of metastatic spread. Myeloma and occasionally a hypernephroma may be indicated by finding a very high ESR. Bone pain from metastic deposits can often be relieved with prostaglandin inhibitors, e.g. indomethacin, but sometimes local radiotherapy is necessary.

Paget's disease may also cause backache, but will be apparent from an X-ray and can be further suspected in the presence of a very high alkaline phosphatase. Most commonly, however, backache is probably a result of soft-tissue disorders which are self-limiting and need treating only with analgesics and support. It must not be forgotten that pain may be referred to the back from an intra-abdominal viscus, e.g. a peptic ulcer, gastric neoplasm, and pancreatitis; that infective conditions occasionally localize into and around the spine; and herpes zoster can present with pain before the rash occurs. Osteomalacia (see p. 67) can also be responsible for back pain, and is diagnosed with the usual radiological and biochemical investigations.

The initial stages in the management of back pain include therefore a careful history, examination of the abdomen as well as the back, and an X-ray of the spine. Laboratory investigation may then be organized on the basis of the radiological and other findings, if any. Should the discomfort persist, especially in the presence of weight loss or other evidence of systemic disease, referral for further investigation is necessary.

CEREBROVASCULAR ACCIDENT

Having confirmed that a patient has suffered a stroke the next decision that must be made is whether or not they should be admitted to hospital. There are undoubtedly many people who have either a minor CVA or adequate home support who can be completely managed at home. Despite this it is the author's opinion that the majority of people with a stroke should be admitted to hospital, at least initially. Domiciliary care can then be resorted to early on if this is appropriate. In a patient in whom domiciliary care is anticipated the following points should be assessed in every case.

Aetiology

This is to ensure there is no treatable underlying cause which could lead to further episodes if not discovered and treated in time. Common cardiovascular conditions include:

Hypertension – but it must be remembered that a mild elevation of blood pressure may be the result and not the cause of the stroke.

Dysrhythmias – which may lower cardiac output and also be responsible for systemic embolization.

Systemic emboli from valvular heart disease, a mural thrombus after a coronary, and large vessel atheroma. Evidence for the latter may be found by listening for a bruit in the neck.

Central nervous system – a tumour or space-occupying lesion will usually produce a gradual or slow onset. Other occasional catches in the elderly include Todd's paralysis after an epileptic attack, a subdural haematoma and less frequently meningitis. The patient's history of epilepsy may not have been known, and the fit may not have been witnessed. In theory a subdural haematoma should have fluctuating signs, but this is not always the case. The presence of meningism and a fever will usually indicate the possibility of meningitis, although blood in the cerebrovascular space produces a similar clinical picture.

Temporal arteritis – this occasionally presents with localizing neurological signs and should be suspected if the appropriate history can be elicited or the patient is known to have a high ESR.

Diabetes mellitus – both hypo- and hyperglycaemia may be associated with localizing neurological signs and indicate the need for attention to the underlying problem.

It can therefore be seen that there are a sufficient number of treatable underlying precipitating factors to warrant the admission of many patients with a stroke to hospital, even if the disability is in itself not an adequate reason for this. In any patient in whom domiciliary care was initially considered, the presence or suspicion of one of these conditions, or of any other condition that has not been mentioned but which is in itself treatable, should lead to hospital referral unless it is considered that the time has come for the patient to be allowed to die gracefully and with dignity at home. Even this decision can be fraught with danger, however, since many patients recover when expected not to do so, and failure to direct prompt attention to the underlying illness, or later on to organize rehabilitation early enough in the recovery phase, may lead to a greater degree of eventual dependency.

Determine the site of the lesion

Cerebrovascular damage in the elderly commonly occurs in the region of the *internal capsule*. Through this structure pass motor fibres, the majority to the other side of the body but in the case of those muscle groups with bilateral innervation, namely the trunk, limb girdles, and neck, to the ipsilateral side also. Sensory and autonomic fibres are also present in the internal capsule and lead to the sensory abnormalities and disturbance of autonomic function in the affected limbs. Fibres connecting with the extrapyramidal system are also present and it may be that damage to these is partly responsible for the alteration in tone and eventual onset of spasticity. Fibres from the optic radiation pass through the lateral wing producing a homonymous field defect, often a full hemianopia.

If the *cerebral cortex* is involved there will be flaccid weakness affecting flexor and extensor muscle groups equally, whereas in the internal capsule lesion there is usually hypertonicity of the flexors and abductors in the arms and of the extensors in the legs. Other indications of a cortical lesion are the typical picture of cortical sensory loss and speech problems, especially dysphasia.

A lesion in the *brain stem* will produce multiple signs because of the large number of vital structures crowded together in a small space. It is usually manifested by the involvement of cranial nerve nuclei affecting the ipsilateral side, since these fibres tend to cross high in the brain stem, and contralateral weakness in the limbs. Evidence of cerebellar involvement or vertigo also indicates a brain-stem territory lesion. Pontine haemorrhage should be suspected in a deeply unconscious patient with bilateral paralysis, small pupils, and a pyrexia. (Small pupils may also be caused by opiates and anticholinergic eye drops as used in glaucoma, and it is possible to be caught out by one of these if the possibility is not considered.)

It is necessary to identify the site of the lesion because of the relevance of this to the prognosis. Brain-stem lesions in particular have a poor prognosis.

Consider the potential prognosis

In an individual patient it is often very difficult to know at the beginning what the outcome is going to be. In general, however, there are many points which may influence the outcome, and these include the site of the lesion as discussed above; the patient's conscious level – since the prognosis is worse in non-haemmorrhagic lesions if the patient is unconscious; the functional level – since the outlook is better the greater the functional level initially; aphasia – since the absence of this indicates a favourable outlook; and parietal lobe damage – which is usually associated with poor functional recovery. In addition one needs to take into account the associated diseases, including those which might precipitate a further cerebrovascular event and those which may cause morbidity in their own right.

Further management

In the acute phase it is also necessary carefully to assess those factors which may prejudice the patient's survival, including the swallowing reflex and the state of hydration. Later, i.e. during the recovery period, it is important to check the following regularly: (i) urinary and faecal incontinence; (ii) pressure sores; (iii) deep venous thrombosis and pulmonary emboli; (iv) constipation; (v) hypostatic pneumonia, and (vi) contractures.

In theory these are all treatable or preventable sequelae and should be attended to as appropriate. It may well be necessary to refer the patient to a geriatric clinic for consideration of additional rehabilitation, e.g. through the day hospital, after the acute phase is over and the patient has begun to return to normal life.

Finally, it is important to note that there is no objective evidence for any benefit in the long term following a completed stroke from the prescription of anticoagulants, aspirin, dipyridamole, dextran, or steroids. Each of these may be of prophylactic benefit in certain situations, e.g. anticoagulation in the presence of mitral stenosis and atrial fibrillation, but it is unlikely to affect a stroke which has already occurred.

Useful advice for old people and their relatives

Coping with dysphasia

1. Talk a little more slowly than normal.
2. Use short sentences of simple construction but not childish language.
3. Avoid 'either . . . or' questions, try to ask questions which require yes and no.
4. Do not rush to finish sentences or supply words.
5. Supplement the spoken word with mime, for example pointing to the object discussed or miming drinking a cup of tea. Try using drawings and pictures of everyday objects for the patient to point to.
6. Remember that the patient can often understand much more than he can say. Do not discuss sensitive matters in front of him.
7. Put important instructions in writing.
8. Ask the advice of the speech therapists if the patient is in hospital or attends day hospital.

CONFUSION

It is often very difficult to be certain whether an elderly person is confused, or merely suffering from loss of memory for recent events, since the latter may masquerade as the former. The opposite is also true of course in many cases, and many an old person has thought to be 'aging' when they have really been showing the initial signs of a dementia. One of the most important steps to take is to confirm whether or not the mental impairment is likely to be caused by a dementing illness, and unfortunately many of the existing mental test scores are unhelpful since they rely upon memory only. Dementia is a global impairment of intellectual ability, and it is important also to test for other parameters. Examples of this are temporal and parietal lobe function, including aphasia, e.g. pointing to a watch and asking what it is called, and then something a little more difficult like the watch strap and then the hand. This will indicate the presence of motor aphasia whilst an indication of receptive problems can be ascertained from enquiring into the function of common domestic articles. Parietal lobe abnormalities can be elicited by asking the patient to raise their right or left hand, to touch their left knee with their right hand, or vice versa, to identify a coin or small object held in the hand, and to draw a square or a clock face. This is a much more sensitive way of ascertaining the presence of a dementing illness than merely relying upon a memory test.

It is also important to mention at this point that the psuedodementia of depression must always be considered if there are other signs indicating the possibility of a depressive illness.

There are two common clinical situations which arise, namely acute confusional states, and the person who exhibits a more chronic course in his or her intellectual impairment. Although there is much overlap between the two, they are probably best considered separately from a purely practical point of view.

Acute confusional states

The commonest cause is undoubtedly infection, especially of the respiratory or urinary tract. Endocrine and metabolic abnormalities are often responsible, including hyperglycaemia, hypoglycaemia, drugs, (especially antiparkinsonian agents, hypnotics, sedatives, and antidepressants), nutritional deficiencies, especially B_{12} and possibly folate, and abnormalities of the urea and electrolytes. Two of these categories, namely myxoedema and nutritional deficiencies, tend to have a slower onset of action than is normally considered classical of an acute confusional state, but on occasions have been noted to present with an apparently rapid onset. This may be because the patient has deteriorated without it being noted until some event makes it more apparent.

Other causes include a cerebrovascular accident, a subdural haematoma, an intracerebral space-occupying lesion, a non-metastatic effect of neoplasm of the bronchus, and other physical problems, such as cardiac and respiratory failure.

It is important also to bear in mind the other causes of a more chronic dementing illness since as mentioned earlier, these can apparently have an acute onset because of the way in which the problem presents.

The initial step in diagnosis is to exclude infection in the usual way, to check a patient's drugs and relate the onset of confusion to the duration of drug

28 *Management of common problems in the elderly*

therapy, and then to screen for the other conditions, e.g. with the aid of a blood-sugar level, urea and electrolyte estimation, B_{12} and folate assay, thyroid function tests, haemoglobin, white count and ESR, and any other investigation that seems appropriate as a result of the history and examination. If a cause is not found, or an illness is encountered which cannot be successfully treated at home, early referral to the geriatric service is necessary.

Chronic confusion/dementia

This can be caused by those conditions already described under the heading of acute confusional states. However, if it has genuinely been present for six months or so it is far more likely that the patient has an irreversible condition such as multiple infarct dementia or more commonly senile Alzheimer's disease. Despite this it is always necessary to exclude the treatable conditions, rectification of which may lead to an improvement in the patient's mental abilities, although often the best that one can hope for is that the progress of the dementia will be arrested or retarded.

Senile Alzheimer's disease is identical with that in the presenile dementia group, and is probably the commonest cause of senile dementia. The other most commonly occurring condition is multi-infarct dementia, i.e. mental impairment resulting from progression of small strokes. In theory, this condition is more likely if the deterioration has been step-wise rather than gradual, the patient has a history of hypertension, or there is evidence of vascular disease elsewhere. It is not always possible, however, to rely upon this evidence and indeed not infrequently multiple-infarct dementia and senile Alzheimer's disease exist together. Both these conditions in life are only diagnosable by exclusion, since brain biopsy, although formerly practised in some circumstances, is clearly unethical at the present time and probably particularly so in the elderly.

Other conditions which must be considered as a potential cause of chronic intellectual impairment, and which should be excluded, are the subdural haematoma, neurosyphilis, parkinsonism, low-pressure hydrocephalus, drug side-effects, myxoedema, and B_{12} deficiency, as well as the other factors mentioned under the heading of the acute confusional state.

The investigations can usually be organized without hospital referral and should include: (i) biochemistry – urea and electrolytes, biochemical screen, especially liver function tests and bone biochemistry, and a blood sugar; (ii) full blood count and ESR; (iii) B_{12} and folate levels; (iv) thyroid function tests, i.e. T4/TSH; (v) WR; (vi) chest and skull X-rays; (vii) MSU; and (viii) other investigations indicated by the history or examination.

If a treatable cause is found then further action would depend upon the nature of the underlying condition. If, as can often be the case, one is no further forward in terms of discovering a potentially treatable lesion, the patient should be referred to the geriatric or psychogeriatric service. In general, ambulant demented patients are probably best referred to the psychiatrist unless further investigations, e.g. a lumbar puncture and/or an isotope or CT scan are considered necessary.

DYSPHAGIA

This is another condition which must be considered seriously in the elderly, but it is often difficult to interpret since many of our elders have only a vague idea of what they are actually complaining of. It is rarely psychogenic in origin and should always be considered carefully. Repeated strokes resulting in a bulbar palsy are thought by some geriatricians to be the commonest cause, but other neurological abnormalities can also occur, as they can in younger people too. Unless one can confidently diagnose a neurological abnormality, any patient in whom dysphagia presents should be allowed the benefit of the doubt and a barium swallow organized. Although a neoplastic lesion in the stomach (usually the fundus) or oesophagus may be revealed, other conditions may occasionally surprise one. Found not that infrequently are oesophageal pouches or diverticula, strictures of a benign nature, and occasionally reflux oesophagitis associated with a hiatus hernia – particularly if it is of the sliding variety. Systemic sclerosis, although it does not feature prominently amongst the causes of dysphagia, is more prevalent amongst the elderly.

The Plummer–Vinson syndrome is usually found in women after long-standing iron deficiency. It is due to a postcricoid web, but the iron deficiency must have been present for a considerable period before the diagnosis can be entertained, and even then a barium swallow is necessary before the diagnosis can be confirmed.

Treatment

The nature of the treatment depends upon the underlying lesion, e.g. it may be possible periodically to dilate a 'simple' stricture, but a malignant obstruction will need surgical intervention of a more drastic nature if the patient is fit enough, or a palliative procedure such as the insertion of a tube. A surgical approach may also be necessary in some of the other conditions, but if the cause is neurological it may be necessary to resort to a long-term nasogastric tube, with all the attendant problems.

ERYTHROCYTE SEDIMENTATION RATE

The erythrocyte sedimentation rate is often higher in older people than is considered normal in younger patients. Even a fall of 50 mm an hour has been accepted as normal by some authorities. At this level, however, careful consideration is necessary before dismissing it as a normal expression of aging. It is not uncommon in older people to find an ESR up to or even above thirty mm per hour and this is where most of the difficulties of interpretation arise. This is especially true since there are so many other variables which affect the ESR and some of which are likely to be present in many of the elderly. These include the haemoglobin level itself and cardiac failure. In addition to this, technical factors also play a role in accelerating the rate of fall and perhaps one of the commonest of these is failing to ensure that the sedimentation tube is absolutely vertical. A deviation of a mere five degrees from the vertical can double the sedimentation rate.

If the elevated ESR is the only abnormal finding and the remainder of the laboratory investigations are normal and the history and examination unremarkable, it is not unreasonable to wait a short while and repeat it after a week or two. If the original value was spurious or due to a passing subclinical infection, it is likely that the result would have returned to normal. On the contrary, cryptic pathology previously present may have progressed to a point where it will declare itself on reassessment. Persistent elevation of the sedimentation rate requires further investigation.

If the ESR is very high, e.g. a 100 or over, it is important to consider first the possibility of neoplastic disease, such as a neoplasm with secondary spread, a hypernephroma with or without secondaries, and also multiple myeloma, as well as non-malignant conditions, in particular the collagenoses. The history will indicate whether or not temporal arteritis and other related conditions, e.g. polymyalgia rheumatica are a possibility. This can also cause the ESR to be very high. Appropriate investigations will indicate whether any of the other conditions mentioned are likely to be responsible.

The conditions mentioned above must also be considered if the ESR is elevated, but not as high as a 100. In addition to the appropriate investigations for these conditions, it is also necessary to arrange for routine urea and electrolytes and biochemical screen, an MSU, a full blood count and film, and if appropriate sputum for culture and microscopy. The presence of occult blood in the stool should be sought, and may indicate GI tract pathology. Cryptic infection, such as tuberculosis and subacute bacterial endocarditis, are occasionally responsible and should be considered if no other cause is discovered. It is also important to remember that the elevated ESR associated with rheumatoid arthritis may persist for a long time after the joint disease has become extinguished, but one must not assume this to be responsible for an elevated ESR unless any other coexistent pathologies have been excluded.

Occasionally a low erythrocyte sedimentation rate is discovered in an older person. It does not usually present a problem and is more commonly associated with polycythaemia, hyperviscosity states caused by other diseases, and congestive cardiac failure.

The erythrocyte sedimentation rate is very non-specific and has little diagnostic significance. It is, however, helpful in alerting one that all is not well, and also when following the progress of a disease or its treatment.

FALLS

Falls in the elderly should never be allowed to pass without consideration of their aetiology. It is easy to hear about an older person falling and just allow it to pass through one's mind without registering. However, the investigation of falls can often lead to worthwhile preventive medicine. It is very difficult to present a succinct account of the potential underlying conditions since these are so legion. Instead, a practical approach is described which concentrates on the commoner causes, and those for which it is possible to take some action. In general, the history and examination are more helpful than investigation, which less frequently indicate a cause other than something which has been suspected already.

Although there is no substitute for a full history and examination system by system, there are four points of particular importance which should be sought during the history. These are as follows.

Vertigo

Many older people have great difficulty in accurately describing vertigo, giddiness, dizziness, etc. Falls are infrequently caused by true vertigo, but when this situation does arise it is important to exclude wax in the external auditory meatus before looking for more complex conditions, such as brain-stem lesions and damage secondary to drug therapy. These will be responsible for only a few cases in older people, as also is Menières disease, a diagnosis with which many people are mislabelled.

An association between dizziness or giddiness and change in head position, e.g. extension such as when looking up to a high cupboard or lateral rotation as in looking both ways before crossing the road, indicates the possibility of cervical spondylosis and vertebrobasilar insufficiency.

Accident hazards

The commonest cause of falls is probably the accident hazard. Many minor falls of this nature are not reported to the doctor unless trauma ensues. Common hazards include inadequate lighting, especially on staircases, loose mats, and trailing electric cables. These are common findings in the homes of the elderly.

Loss of consciousness

This is best confirmed from a reliable witness.

Relation to posture

Postural hypotension occurs more commonly than is generally realized and should be directly questioned for, and the blood pressure tested in the lying and erect positions in all people who have a history of falling. A drop in systolic pressure of 20 mm of mercury or more is usually significant, especially if associated with symptoms. When present, the following underlying conditions

32 Management of common problems in the elderly

need to be excluded; hypokalaemia, evidence of autonomic dysfunction and its possible causes, e.g. tabes and diabetes mellitus, and drug side-effects. Drugs that are particularly likely to be responsible include antidepressants, antiparkinsonian drugs, hypotensive agents, hypnotics, and diuretics. These can all aggravate or precipitate postural hypotension which is then best treated by removing the cause. This should be followed where necessary by prescribing elastic stockings, but if it is difficult for the elderly person in question to put these on, stockingette of the tubigrip type may be very helpful. Finally, small doses of fludrocortisone may help in difficult cases. If after these measures there has been no improvement in the postural hypotension, further investigation is usually necessary and this is best carried out in a hospital outpatient setting.

One practical point of help is to counsel the patient to stand up or change his position slowly, and pause until the giddiness passes off. In many people this may obviate the need for elastic stockings or fludrocortisone.

The major systems will now be considered in turn:

Cardiovascular system

If the falls are preceded or accompanied by palpitations, an ECG and in many cases a 24-hour ambulatory tape are necessary in order to exclude a dysrhythmia. Falls may also be a consequence of a Stokes–Adams attack, or an episode of bradycardia, and once again an ECG and a 24-hour tape are necessary in order to substantiate the diagnosis. Since both brady- and tachyarrhythmias may be symptomless apart from the falls, and often only occur sporadically, the standard ECG on its own is frequently unhelpful. For this reason any patient who has an unexplained history of falls should be considered a candidate for 24-hour monitoring unless this is inappropriate for other reasons.

Central nervous system

The majority of falls probably originate because of an abnormality somewhere in the central nervous system. Cervical spondylosis has already been mentioned, and a cervical collar may be helpful in some people. Unfortunately, degenerative arthritis in the neck is present in so many elderly people without any symptoms and is often an incidental finding in someone with a history of falling.

Disturbance of posterior-column function, in particular because of B_{12} deficiency and syphilis, will lead to impaired proprioception and a greater tendency to fall. Therefore, if joint position sense is found to be defective, it is essential to estimate the serum B_{12} and a WR. Occasionally, impaired joint position sense is found to occur as part of a more generalized peripheral neuropathy, in which case it is important to exclude B_1 deficiency as well as B_{12}, diabetes mellitus, and also to consider the following conditions which occasionally occur in elderly patients as a cause of peripheral neuropathy – drugs and alcohol, lead poisoning (especially older houses with lead pipes in soft water districts), carcinomatosis, and amyloid.

More commonly than peripheral neuropathy, extrapyramidal symptoms, i.e.

parkinsonism, are implicated. Before treating with antiparkinsonian drugs it is first necessary to ensure that the symptoms are not iatrogenic in nature. Phenothiazines, e.g. chlorpromazine and thioridazine are the commonest offenders and occasionally a buterophenone, e.g. haloperidol is also responsible. Under these circumstances treatment is best initiated by withdrawing the offending drug. If it is not possible to do this for any reason, an anticholinergic/antiparkinsonian preparation should be prescribed, i.e. benzhexol or orphenadrine, rather than an L-dopa combination preparation. It is the rigidity and the bradykinesia which contribute most to falls, and these are probably best treated with an L-dopa preparation if the parkinsonism is not drug induced. Whenever prescribing these drugs one must bear in mind the possible side-effects that can occur.

Cerebellar ataxia most commonly results from cerebrovascular disease in older people and is occasionally responsible for, or contributes to, falling. Cerebellar dysfunction may also be produced by drugs, especially phenytoin, barbiturates, and alcohol, and occasionally by lesions in the cerebellopontine angle, e.g. an acoustic neuroma. A patient with cerebellar ataxia is best referred for further investigation, since occasionally a treatable cause is responsible, but it is worth withdrawing the drugs first if it is thought these may be implicated.

Epilepsy also causes falls and sometimes if the fits are not witnessed, the patient is found on the floor and the epileptic nature of the incidence goes unrecognized. In old people living alone this can happen quite frequently without the diagnosis being considered. It is important to remember that epilepsy in older people may well be due to an old cerebrovascular accident scar, but can also result from space-occupying lesions and metabolic rather than physical causes. The onset of epilepsy in an older person should result in referral for further investigation and management.

There are other causes of falls due to abnormalities in the nervous system and these include poor eyesight, e.g. due to a cataract–extraction may well improve the situation, transient ischaemic attacks and early dementia. The latter two are difficult to treat, but it is occasionally worth prescribing an aspirin tablet b.d. for someone with TIAs if there is no contra-indication and no other obvious cause for the attack. As yet, however, there is no objective evidence that this is effective.

Musculoskeletal system

Arthritis is the commonest cause of, or contributory factor to, falls as far as abnormalities of the musculoskeletal system are concerned. Osteoarthrosis, and occasionally rheumatoid arthritis with or without associated osteoarthrosis are the types of arthritis that are most usually involved, but there are other conditions and it is important not to forget that diabetes and syphilis may be responsible for a grossly disorganized painless joint. An X-ray of the joint, especially if compared to the 'normal' side will help establish the diagnosis. This is worthwhile since chronological age on its own is not a contra-indication to standard surgical management and an accurate diagnosis is in any case necessary to justify medical treatment.

It is often forgotten that disease of the muscles themselves may contribute to a tendency to fall. Most commonly this takes the form of a proximal myopathy such is found in thyrotoxicosis, Cushing's disease (which is rare in older patients), osteomalacia, electrolyte abnormalities, and carcinoma (especially of the bronchus). Any of these conditions, if considered, can be diagnosed with the usual laboratory investigations which can be arranged from the general practice setting. Occasionally, severe wasting of the quadriceps in a patient who has been in bed for a long time is difficult to differentiate from a proximal myopathy, but in the latter other muscle groups, including those of the upper limb girdle are often also affected.

Just occasionally, a diabetic amyotrophy is responsible. This affects men more than women and is associated with wasting of the thigh muscles, and severe pain.

Drugs

Falls are often iatrogenic since many drugs may contribute to a tendency in this direction, especially if they affect the conscious level, e.g. hypnotics, sedatives, and antidepressants. Those causing postural hypotension have already been mentioned.

If the list of conditions described above can be excluded and the patient continues to fall, referral to a geriatrician is advisable.

The management of instability

Even after careful assessment and treatment many old people continue to be either at risk of falling, are afraid of falling, or both, and they and their relatives need help to cope at home. They need information about the factors which put their elderly relative at risk of falling, support and reassurance if they are very anxious, and involvement in the promotion of exercise and the use of walking aids, and preparation for a fall.

The promotion of exercise and confidence.

The person who is afraid of falling may enter a vicious cycle.

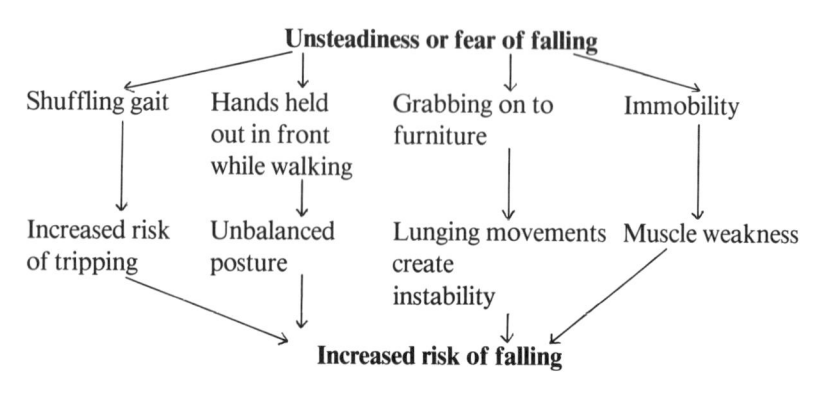

Unsteadiness or fear of falling

Shuffling gait	Hands held out in front while walking	Grabbing on to furniture	Immobility
↓	↓	↓	↓
Increased risk of tripping	Unbalanced posture	Lunging movements create instability	Muscle weakness

Increased risk of falling

The promotion of exercises and the re-education of the patient are therefore of vital importance. The best approach is for a physiotherapist to pay a home visit to work with the old person and his relatives, but this is often difficult to arrange and visits to day hospital for physiotherapy have to be used as a basis for educating the patient and relatives.

The old person should be encouraged to: stand up straight; lift her feet and step out; walk slowly and steadily. There is also evidence that any form of exercise helps restore proprioceptive fitness, the promotion of exercise and confidence to go hand in hand.

The provision of walking aids (see p. 48)

Proper preparation for a fall
If it seems likely that the old person will fall, a number of measures can be suggested to minimize the risk of harmful consequences:

The old person should be taught how to rise from the ground. It is possible to teach people who are considerably disabled how to rise, for example the hemiplegic patient can be taught how to use his strong side to best advantage by a physiotherapist.

Arrangements should be made so that the old person can call for help if he cannot rise, either by the provision of a telephone, or by asking neighbours to be prepared to notice a code or signal, such as three taps on the wall, or to call if the curtains are not opened.

By making all parts of the house as warm as possible the risk of hypothermia can be avoided.

HEARING LOSS

The threshold for hearing deteriorates from the 30s onwards and there are other changes which can be demonstrated in the normal physiology of hearing as age progresses. From a practical point of view, however, it is probably necessary to take seriously a person's complaint of deafness if they are having difficulty hearing normal conversations, and they can probably be definitively diagnosed as suffering from mild impairment if they are unable to interpret speech when a slightly louder voice than that employed in normal conversation is used.

The first step is to look in the ear and see whether there is a significant degree of wax in the external auditory meatus. If the deafness persists after this has been removed, testing with a tuning fork will quickly indicate whether it has a conductive or sensory-neural basis. If bone conduction (when the tuning fork is placed on the mastoid process behind the ear) is better than air, then a conduction loss is present. Occasionally this is due to conditions such as otitis media and otosclerosis in the elderly, and the appropriate symptoms should be sought in the history. Unfortunately, sensory-neural loss is commoner in older people and is rarely attributable to an underlying condition, and it is therefore not very often that one can treat a patient successfully. There is mixed opinion as to whether vascular disease on its own can lead to deafness of this type, but in theory it is possible. Other potential causes include drugs, especially streptomycin and quinine, and Menière's disease. Again appropriate information to indicate these possibilities will be elicited from the history.

Help for the hard of hearing

The elderly person who is hard of hearing needs considerable help and encouragement. A number of aids and services are available to help people who are hard of hearing, and a check-list is given below:

Telephone adaptations to allow the person to hear the phone ringing and conversation – leaflets and advice from the local telephone exchange.

Induction loop for television reception allowing the deaf person to receive amplified sound.

Flashing lights instead of the door-bell.

Ear trumpets.

Hearing aids, which should never be bought privately, except on the advice of the staff of the local NHS Hearing Aid Clinic.

However, these aids are only fully effective if the person is given support and help when using them. The best means of producing support and helping the person adapt to the loss of hearing is to introduce him to a club organized by the Social Worker for the deaf. In large towns and cities there are separate deaf and hard of hearing clubs, but in small towns it is more common for a single deaf and hard of hearing club to exist. These clubs are excellent rehabilitation centres and the deaf person can obtain all the information about aids and services in addition to advice on lip reading and the maintenance of his aid. However, many people are reluctant to acknowledge that they are having increasing difficulty with hearing, and relatives need to be involved.

Advice for relatives

Relatives are as much in need of advice as deaf people. They need to be told not only about the range of aids and services available, but also how they can help the person who has difficulty with hearing. This advice can be summarized in a list of dos and don'ts.

Do	**Don't**
Face the light (and be sure there is sufficient light, artificial if needs be)	Mumble your words
Speak clearly and naturally	Exaggerate your lip movements
Sit or stand within two metres of your relative. Experiment until you find out how close you should sit or stand to make his hearing aid or lip reading useful	Put your hand over your mouth when talking

Do	**Don't**
Look directly at your relative when speaking to him	Shout
Be friendly, casual, and tolerant	Smoke during your conversation
Have sympathetic understanding, but not pity	Say one word over and over again, change the wording, and try again. Many words are difficult to see on the lips
Be patient with mistakes	Wear dark glasses. Much can be said by your eyes
Watch for signs of fatigue	Allow the deaf person to become isolated: seek the advice of the Social Worker for the deaf if you feel he is becoming withdrawn
Write 'key' words on a pad (especially proper names) when necessary	
Encourage your relative to attend a club for the deaf or hard of hearing	
Encourage him to seek help if he finds his hearing-aid difficult to use or useless	

Deafness and mental health

Deafness is associated with certain types of mental illness in old age:
   Anxiety.
   Depression.
   Paranoid delusions, sometimes with auditory hallucinations related to tinnitus.
   Confusion, due to the sensory deprivation.
   It is therefore essential to consider the contributions which deafness could be making when an elderly patient presents with one of these symptoms. Furthermore clinical suspicion and questioning may not reveal a significant impairment in hearing. One recent study found that 60 per cent out of a sample of 253 people over the age of 70 had impaired hearing when assessed by pure-tone audiometry which is twice the prevalence found by studies which relied on clinical assessment or self reporting.

HYPERCALCAEMIA

Many an elevated plasma calcium is factitious being the result of stasis of the blood in the vein after a tourniquet has been applied. It is therefore necessary to repeat a calcium estimation in a fasting cuffless sample and also to correct the result in proportion to the serum albumin level. In the elderly three conditions in particular cause a rise in the plasma calcium. Probably the commonest is a neoplasm, especially bronchial carcinoma which can produce a parathormone-like substance. The next commonest cause is probably carcinomatosis associated with multiple osteolytic deposits and may be due to myeloma, a solid tumour, or a lymphoma. The third condition is hyperparathyroidism, but occurs less frequently than the others. A neoplasm may often be suspected on the basis of the findings from the history and the examination in conjunction with a routine blood count, ESR, biochemical screen, and a chest X-ray. Where appropriate, other investigations are necessary such as sputum cytology if a bronchial neoplasm is likely and an MSU to exclude the presence of red blood cells in the case of a hypernephroma. Other evidence indicating the presence of a neoplasm includes an elevated alkaline phosphatase, typical lesions on a skeletal X-ray, and multiple filling defects on a liver scan.

The presence of an elevated plasma calcium level with a decreased fasting plasma phosphate should lead one to consider the possibility of hyperparathyroidism. Additional evidence is also required before this diagnosis can be confirmed, the most important being of course estimating the serum parathormone level through the regional or supraregional assay service. It is, however, often helpful to undertake additional tests before estimating the parathormone level if this is difficult to obtain. An increased urinary calcium and phosphate excretion should also be found in a case of hyperparathyroidism, and a five day course of corticosteroids will usually lower the calcium level in most conditions that cause hypercalcaemia, but not when it is due to hyperparathyroidism.

Other causes of hypercalcaemia include Paget's disease of the bone if the patient is bed-ridden or otherwise immobilized and less frequently vitamin D intoxication or a milk-alkali syndrome. These can usually be screened out on the basis of an adequate history, although it maybe necessary to take this from a third person. There are of course other conditions causing hypercalcaemia such as sarcoid and thyrotoxicosis, but although they occur in the elderly they are an uncommon cause of hypercalcaemia.

Correction factor for plasma calcium level

Adjust calcium level by 0.02 mmol/l for every 1 g/l deviation in total plasma protein level from the reference value of 72 g/l.

HYPERGLYCAEMIA

Although many elderly people have a raised renal threshold for glucose, the upper limit of normal for the blood sugar level is the same as in younger people. The increase in renal threshold will often allow them to run a plasma glucose level that is higher than normal without sugar spilling into the urine and being detected there. This does not mean that the elevated glucose level is acceptable and any elevation in the blood sugar must be considered pathological even if the raised renal threshold is protecting the patient from the effects of fluid and salt loss.

A glucose level two hours after a meal is an effective screening test for diabetes mellitus in the elderly, and if the glucose level is greater than 10 mmol/l, this diagnosis is almost certain. It can be further confirmed by measuring a fasting glucose and detecting glycosuria in many patients. Reflectance meters have made it easier to undertake these measurements in the home. Although a glucose tolerance test is unnecessary in many elderly people, it is sometimes required in the instance of a difficult or borderline case. All glucose estimations should be performed on a blood sample which has been placed in a fluoride tube. It is not widely appreciated that red cell glycolysis may lower the sugar level by as much as a half if left in an unfluoridated tube at room temperature for as little as three hours.

Many elderly diabetics do not need hospital referral since the diagnosis can easily be made within the general practice setting. In a patient in whom the diagnosis has been confirmed, it is important to assess whether there are any complications, for example diabetic retinopathy or cataracts, peripheral vascular disease, coronary artery disease, or proteinurea indicating the possibility of diabetic nephropathy. The neuropathy of diabetes often seems to escape notice possibly because the symptoms or signs are attributed to normal senescence. It should always be searched for and suspicion of its presence should be heightened in the presence of trophic lesions in the feet. Diabetes also causes an autonomic neuropathy in many people which is most usually evident as postural hypotension and bladder or bowel problems.

Before treating a patient for an elevated blood sugar it is important to exclude other factors which may aggravate any hyperglycaemic tendency. These include drugs, especially some diuretics, corticosteroids and perphenazine in addition to other medical conditions, such as Cushing's disease, acromegaly, obesity, and thyrotoxicosis. With the exception of obesity and the drugs, the other conditions are of course rare. If one of these factors is discovered, appropriate treatment may well make it unnecessary to treat the blood sugar itself.

The majority of elderly people with diabetes can be managed with a diet and an oral hypoglycaemic agent. Unfortunately, it is very difficult to encourage the elderly to lose weight as food is so often one of the few pleasures left in their life. Sulphonylureas are usually the drugs of first choice, but it is probably best to avoid chlorpropamide since this has a long half-life and is excreted by the kidney. Renal impairment is commoner in the elderly and also in the presence of diabetes and dangerous levels of chlorpropamide may build up in the circulation. Unless renal function is known to be normal it is probably best to use one of the shorter acting sulphonylureas. These, however, stimulate insulin secretion which may induce hunger and overeating and result in an increase in weight.

The problem of lactic acidosis associated with the prescription of biguanides is well known and is particularly likely to occur in patients with hepatic and renal impairment, especially in the presence of tissue anoxia, such as is associated with cardiogenic shock. Lactic acidosis may occur nevertheless despite the absence of these factors. Phenformin is probably best avoided where possible.

Insulin is needed in surprisingly few elderly diabetics, but when it is necessary to prescribe this, the principles of treatment are the same as in younger people. Failing eyesight and arthritic hands make it difficult for many an older person to administer their own insulin and it may well be necessary to train relatives or friends to administer it, or ask the district nurse to do it instead.

Any diabetic in whom control of the blood sugar is difficult to achieve, and it must be remembered that hypoglycaemia is as dangerous as hyperglycaemia, or in whom there are complications is probably best referred to hospital for assessment, even though the subsequent management may well be left in the hands of the general practitioner.

Ketonuria

Ketonuria indicates diabetic keto-acidosis if glycosuria is also present, and should be treated appropriately. Severe vomiting will also lead to ketonuria, but in the absence of glycosuria. In addition, starvation, or fasting such as occurs during enforced bed rest in a person living on their own, may also lead to ketonuria. Treatment of the underlying illness and appropriate support will usually remedy the situation.

HYPOALBUMINAEMIA

Albumin levels are often a little lower in older than younger people without there being any pathological reason for this. When an old person becomes ill, however, the albumin often sinks to an even lower level, apparently because of the general debilitating effects of the illness. Despite this a low serum albumin can be caused by a specific condition and these must be considered before attributing hypoalbuminaemia to either age or a general effect of an illness.

The causes of a low albumin are legion, but as usual the history and examination may well be helpful. Amongst the commoner causes are malabsorption and an inadequate dietary intake, when supportive evidence will be found from a routine blood film and biochemistry, such as a macrocytic or microcytic anaemia, or the biochemical concomitants of osteomalacia. If a gastro-intestinal tract pathology is suspected from the patient's symptoms, amongst the commoner causes of a protein-losing gastroenteropathy are neoplasia, hypertrophic gastritis, Crohn's disease, and ulcerative colitis. Barium studies that can be arranged on an outpatient basis will often reveal the underlying pathology, but it may be necessary to refer the patient on to hospital for other procedures, such as endoscopy.

Liver disease is also a cause of a low serum albumin and if so there will often be other stigmata of hepatic pathology and derangement of the liver function tests. Protein loss from the renal tract will also lead to a degree of hypoalbuminaemia, especially if there is a nephrotic syndrome. In general, however, the minor degree of proteinurea found in the urine of many elderly people does not contribute significantly to a low serum albumin. Despite this proteinurea should be considered further in its own right.

Sometimes a low serum albumin is accompanied by a low serum sodium and urea and a low haematocrit indicating the possibility of an expanded plasma volume, caused for example by secondary hyperaldosteronism. If this condition is suspected, it is probably best to refer the patient on to hospital for further investigation.

It is often extremely difficult to know when to investigate further a patient with a low serum albumin. There is a limit to the number of investigations that are reasonable in an older person, particularly when some of them are not going to reveal any treatable underlying pathology. In general, however, having excluded treatable conditions, it is reasonable not to investigate further a patient with a low albumin level unless it is very low (e.g. less than 25 g/l), continuing to fall, or associated with symptoms.

Treatment consists in correcting any underlying aetiological factor since it is not possible to raise the serum albumin by alternative means such as an infusion of albumin. Symptoms may well have to be treated by simple measures, such as elastic stockings for peripheral oedema.

HYPOCALCAEMIA

As mentioned above a low serum calcium in an elderly patient may well merely be a reflection of the serum albumin level. It is therefore necessary to correct for the protein level and a formula is given on p. 38. If a low albumin is detected as the cause for hypocalcaemia the hypoalbuminaemia should be investigated rather than the hypocalcaemia.

One of the most frequent causes of a low serum calcium in an older person is dietary vitamin D deficiency or malabsorption. Under these circumstances osteomalacia is often present and a low calcium will be accompanied by a low serum phosphate and an elevated alkaline phosphatase. This is indicated clinically from the history and additional investigations since the findings on examination are rarely helpful. Amongst the tests that can be employed are the faecal fat estimation and barium studies. The latter will often define any underlying gastro-intestinal cause for malabsorption if this is present.

Coeliac disease is not very common in the elderly but does occur, and if no other cause for malabsorption is found a jejunal biopsy may well be helpful. This would require hospital referral, although the other investigations mentioned up until this point can easily be arranged without sending the patient to hospital.

Chronic renal failure is often associated with resistance to vitamin D, and results in hypocalcaemia. There will usually be other evidence or a past history to indicate the existence of chronic renal failure. The serum alkaline phosphatase and phosphate levels, however, are often unhelpful and maybe either normal or elevated.

Any patient who has undergone previous thyroid surgery must be suspected of having hypoparathyroidism if they present with a low calcium. This is uncommon but is easily missed since the scar is often almost invisible in an older person, and they may well have forgotten their previous thyroid surgery. Acute pancreatitis may also cause hypocalcaemia, but is not a common finding in the elderly. It is often associated also with glycosuria and a plasma amylase level may confirm the diagnosis. This should be checked if a low calcium is accompanied by typical symptoms. As usual one must always consider the drugs that a patient is taking when trying to elucidate the cause of hypocalcaemia. Amongst those most likely to be at fault are anticonvulsants, steroids such as stilboestrol, anabolic steroids, and also carbenoxolone.

HYPOKALAEMIA

The serum potassium level is not a good guide to the potassium balance of the body since this element is found mainly inside the cells and the level in the blood will reflect partly the amount of water in the extracellular and vascular spaces. Potassium leaks out of cells when there is an acidosis, as occurs in renal failure and uncontrolled diabetes, and may produce a high level in the serum which does not reflect an increase in total body potassium. Indeed in the latter condition the body is often in negative potassium balance. Hypokalaemia, however, when accompanied by an alkalosis is always significant and may well be even in the absence of a high bicarbonate. Symptoms of a low potassium include a weak apathetic patient with a tendency to depression or confusion and lack of bowel motility resulting in constipation. Many general practitioners have the facilities to do an ECG, and in the presence of significant potassium depletion there will be flattening or inversion of the T waves with a prominent U wave and a long Q-T interval.

The aetiology of a low body potassium is most conveniently considered in the following order, although each condition should be excluded since there is often more than one reason:

Diet – illness and bed rest often lead to an inadequate diet because of an associated anorexia, or inability to prepare food. The potassium can quickly fall in these circumstances, and if the dietetic history indicates that the previous nutritional status was inadequate hypokalaemia will almost certainly ensue.

Drugs – there are several drugs which will lead to potassium loss. Diuretics are the chief offender, especially some of the combination tablets where there is an inadequate potassium supplement for the diuretic effect of the major component. Amongst the other drugs that cause hypokalaemia those most commonly encountered are carbenoxolone sodium and corticosteroids.

Loss of potassium from the gastrointestinal tract – both diarrhoea and vomiting can cause potassium loss if they are persistent. This is obviously apparent from the history and there will also be signs of dehydration, and an electrolyte estimation may well reveal the loss of other salts. Less commonly, but still an important cause of potassium loss from the bowel is the patient with a history of purgative abuse. This tends to produce larger bulky stools with a high potassium content.

Loss of potassium into the urine – the human kidney appears to have been developed to cope with that period of our evolution when we had a diet high in potassium and low in sodium. It is therefore very competent at conserving sodium and less so potassium. If supra-imposed upon this there is a degree of distal tubular dysfunction, as may occur in pyleonephritis and back pressure from an obstructive uropathy, the potassium conserving ability of the nephron is seriously affected. If one suspects that the potassium is being lost in the urine, a 24-hour collection can easily be carried out in the patient's home and dispatched to the laboratory for estimation. It is probably best to send a complete collection rather than just an aliquot, if this is possible. If this is impossible it is necessary to collect urine for 24 hours into a single container, measuring the potassium concentration in a portion of this rather than sending to the laboratory a specimen obtained at one point in a 24-hour period. The potassium excretion is not necessarily constant throughout the day.

There are of course other causes for a low potassium, but these are less likely to be encountered, or noted in the patient's home environment. Examples are the treatment of a high blood sugar level with insulin, the administration of glucose parentrally and the treatment of a severe anaemia, especially that due to B_{12} or folate deficiency. The aetiology of the hypokalaemia is often obvious from the history, but if the cause remains obscure and the patient has obvious symptoms attributable to hypokalaemia, hospital referral is necessary to exclude the less common causes such as Cushing's syndrome, hyperaldosteronism, etc.

The treatment in the first place is correction if possible of the underlying cause. If potassium replacement is necessary it is best to use a preparation containing potassium chloride since some of the other potassium salts exacerbate the hypochloraemia which often accompanies hypokalaemia. The upper gastro-intestinal tract ulceration which is associated with potassium supplements is well known and is a good reason for avoiding tablets if possible and prescribing instead a liquid preparation for the majority of elderly patients.

A severe hypokalaemia predisposes to cardiac dysrhythmias in addition to the other effects and is probably best treated in hospital with intravenous supplements.

HYPONATRAEMIA

The serum sodium level in the fit elderly is the same as in younger people. However, many ill elderly people have a lower sodium than one would expect. In many instances no underlying cause for this is ever found and it rights itself as their conditions improves.

One of the commonest remediable causes of hyponatraemia is probably sodium loss due to diuretic treatment. This should be suspected in anybody on diuretics, even if they still have significant peripheral oedema. There will often be other evidence of fluid and potassium loss in addition to the hyponatraemia. Under these circumstances, it is necessary to stop or reduce the dose of diuretic if this is possible.

Salt may also be lost from the kidneys as a result of a salt losing nephropathy, such as can occur in the presence of hydronephrosis, pyleonephritis, and possibly nephrosclerosis. This may well be accompanied by proteinuria and other evidence of renal impairment, such as an elevation of the urea and creatinine. In the majority of cases investigation should be limited to excluding remediable causes.

Salt loss from the gastro-intestinal tract may occur in diarrhoea and vomiting and also in patients with intestinal obstruction or a paralytic ileus. These conditions are usually self-evident and appropriate treatment is along the standard lines. If the hyponatraemia is accompanied by hyperkalemia, Addison's disease is a possibility, but this is extremely rare in the elderly. If Addison's disease is suspected, hospital referral is necessary.

Many elderly people have a low sodium as a result of a dilutional effect of water retention. This can occur for a variety of reasons, and possibly most commonly because of a defect in osmoregulation. It has been shown that even many fit elderly people have impaired osmoregulatory capacity. It may also be the result of other factors, for instance the inability of the kidney to excrete sufficient fluid because of poor renal blood flow, as may occur in conditions such as cardiac failure. Inappropriate secretion of antidiuretic hormone is another cause of dilutional hyponatraemia and is known to occur in a multitude of conditions, including malignancy, respiratory conditions including pneumonia and more chronic disorders, head injuries, and as a side-effect of some drug therapy, for instance chlorpopamide. This is best confirmed by measuring the osmolality of the urine when it will be found that the hyponatraemia is associated with an inappropriately high urine osmolality and an elevated sodium content. Under normal circumstances hyponatraemia is associated with a very low urinary sodium as the kidney attempts to conserve the latter. The osmolality could probably be measured by the laboratory from a general practice setting, but if the diagnosis is confirmed, hospital referral for further investigation is probably best.

HYPOTHERMIA

This is defined as a central body temperature which has fallen to below 35°C. It is necessary to measure it with a low-reading rectal thermometer, or using a low-reading thermometer to measure the temperature of a freshly passed specimen of urine. It is a medical emergency and should lead to immediate hospital admission. The survival rate is low and death is precipitated by arrhythmias, metabolic abnormalities especially acidosis, hypoglycaemia, and hypokalaemia among other causes. From the general practice point of view prevention is more important than treatment, and the following factors should routinely be considered in every elderly patient before winter sets in:

1. Exposure to a low environmental temperature, e.g. an unheated and poorly insulated house. This unfortunately is the lot of many of our elders and the grants which can be made available to assist in heating are insufficient, but a person at risk should be put in contact with the Social Worker so they can at least be considered for them (see p. 190 for further discussion).

2. Pre-existing endocrinological abnormalities. Myxoedema and hypopituitarism lead to a fall in the metabolic rate and a greater than average chance of developing hypothermia. This should therefore be borne in mind in any patient who is known to suffer with either of these two hormonal abnormalities.

3. Drugs. Various drugs can precipitate hypothermia either by causing body heat loss by vasodilatation and reducing shivering, or by causing sedation which results in exposure. Those sometimes implicated include chlorpromazine and other phenothiazines, barbiturates, antidepressants and alcohol.

While awaiting ambulance transport, it can be tempting to try and start the re-warming process. This can lead to complications, especially if it results in the body temperature rising at a rate of more than half a degree centigrade an hour. It is therefore best to wrap the patient well with blankets and employ heating to take the chill off the room, rather than at this stage to try and raise the patient's temperature artificially.

IMMOBILITY

Many patients are referred to a geriatric clinic with the diagnosis of 'The Gone off their Legs Syndrome'. In reality this is a very non-specific presentation of disease and underlying aetiological factors, which are often multiple with one being the final precipitating factor, are so legion that it is only possible to give a few basic principles to consider when trying to elucidate the underlying cause.

1. Generalized weakness – this is a common complaint in patients presenting in this way, and although tempting to ascribe this as a non-specific symptom, it may indicate specific underlying abnormalities, including the myopathy of thyrotoxicosis, malignancy, osteomalacia, and other conditions such as polymyalgia rheumatica and not uncommonly electrolyte

abnormalities. Although hypokalaemia is the commonest of the latter, hyponatraemia may also be a contributory factor.

2. Arthritis – osteoarthrosis, and less commonly one of the other arthritic conditions, is commonly a contributory factor. The knees are most frequently involved, but the hip is also a site of predilection (see p. 20).

3. Neurological conditions – there are many potential neurological abnormalities which can result in or aggravate a tendency towards immobility. Probably the commonest include the unsuspected cerebrovascular accident and parkinsonism. A clue to the former is the tendency of the patient always to fall, or be weakest on, one side. Parkinsonism is often drug induced and should be suspected in anybody taking phenothiazines or haloperidol. Less commonly a peripheral neuropathy, such as that due to a neoplasm, B_{12} deficiency or diabetes mellitus may be involved. The other neurological abnormalities are probably best sought for and investigated in a hospital setting.

4. Cardiorespiratory abnormalities – these are usually self-apparent from the symptoms, or examination of the patient and include of course shortness of breath on exertion, chest pain and intermittent claudication.

5. Painful feet – pain in the feet is often tolerated by older people partly because they believe it to be inevitable, partly because they know how difficult it is to obtain NHS chiropody. One common cause of foot problems is the difficulty which some old people have in cutting their toe-nails – 18 per cent of men and 29 per cent of women can only cut their nails with help from others.

Useful advice for old people and their relatives

Cutting toe-nails

1. Do not cut the toe-nails of people with diabetes or vascular disease: seek expert advice.
2. Always cut the toe-nail straight across, soaking the feet in hot water makes cutting easier.
3. Press down the soft tissue on either side of the nail gently five times with a cotton tipped stick, after finishing the nail trimming.
4. If a nail is very thick and heavy rub a nail-file across the surface keeping it flat and being careful not to file the skin.
5. Seek the advice of a district nurse or qualified chiropodist if any part of the foot develops an ulcer, or has a cut which will not heal.
6. Do not try to cut or pare corns with a razor blade.
7. If in doubt ask the advice of the district nurse or a qualified chiropodist.

Useful advice for old people and their relatives

Finding a chiropodist

If the National Health Service chiropodist cannot see an older person whose relatives cannot cope and they have to seek help privately, it is essential to choose a properly qualified chiropodist, that is one with the letters SRch – State Registered Chiropodist or Mchs – Member of the Chiropodial Society, after his name. Social Security cannot pay the fees of private chiropody under any circumstances.

Help is given either by their relatives or a Chiropodist, and because relatives play such an important part in foot care they require simple instruction about the best means of cutting nails safely and how to choose a qualified Chiropodist, if NHS chiropody is unavailable.

6. Others – amongst the other conditions that must always be considered when an old person is off their feet are the early stages of dementia, depression, timor cadendi (fear of falling) in which the cause of the falls is the most important factor to elucidate, minor foot pathologies which are more incapacitating than the doctor appreciates, and last, but not least, unsuspected fractures, especially of the femoral neck.

It can be seen that the majority of these conditions will be apparent after examining the patient and arranging appropriate investigations. Although the diagnosis can often be made at home, the majority of patients who have been off their feet for any length of time are probably best rehabilitated in a hospital setting because they need more intensive physiotherapy and occupational therapy than can be delivered at home, or through a Day Hospital or outpatient setting. It is probably best to refer a patient who has taken to his or her bed to a Geriatrician, probably for a domiciliary visit, earlier rather than later in the course of their illness.

The management of immobility

Even after careful assessment and treatment of the causes of an old person's impairment of mobility, it is often impossible to restore mobility fully, and the old person and his relatives have to be given advice on how to cope with the immobility. A home visit by a Physiotherapist, if it is possible to arrange this, or Domiciliary Occupational Therapist, allows four possibilities to be explored:

Alteration of chair height

Many old people are immobilized because the chair in which they sit is too low. This rarely causes complete immobility, but if mobility is to be encouraged it is essential to make it as easy as possible for the old person to stand up. The Occupational Therapist may:

Teach the old person how to stand up – common mistakes are failure to move the bottom to the front of the chair and failure to position the feet correctly.

Use blocks under the feet or castors on the chair.

Use a high 'geriatric chair'.

Advice on exercise

If not given specific advice on exercise many people will assume that 'rest' is beneficial and will not take sufficient exercise. It is therefore important to give an 'exercise prescription', for example by saying that 'you can improve your health by walking to the back gate at least twice a day'. A physiotherapist may be able to help the elderly person and his family plan an exercise programme, setting goals which make successively greater demands on the person with the mobility problem.

The provision of mobility aids

These should not be given too soon because they very quickly create dependence and can lead to a further loss of fitness, for example the walking frame 'Zimmer' can cause shoulder and spinal stiffness because of the forward lean it requires. Nevertheless mobility aids have a significant contribution to make and the needs of the patient for a mobility aid should always be considered:

A walking frame.

Rails, either up the stairs or along the hall.

Rails at front and back steps or handles beside single steps.

A wheelchair.

If blindness is the cause of the immobility the advice of the Mobility Officer for the Blind should be sought.

Adaption of the dwelling

The domiciliary occupational therapist can assess the need for:

A stair lift.

Ramps at the front or back door.

The installation of a downstairs toilet or bathroom.

Relatives should be advised never to undertake the expense of major alterations without the advice of the domiciliary occupational therapists.

INCONTINENCE OF FAECES

This usually occurs for one of three major reasons:

1. Secondary to large bowel pathology, or diarrhoea from any cause.

2. Secondary to faecal impaction when it is often associated with incontinence of urine as mentioned in the following section. This will not

always be apparent on rectal examination because the impaction can occur higher than the finger can feel, in which case if suspected from palpating the descending colon, a plain abdominal film is necessary.

3. Secondary to neurological damage.

The presence of large bowel disease or diarrhoea can usually be ascertained from the history, and the findings on examination. Whether or not further action is necessary depends upon the underlying pathology. If a local cause is discovered, however, appropriate treatment may be helpful, but in practice the response is often disappointing. Despite this, an attempt should be made, wherever feasible, to rectify an underlying condition.

Faecal impaction occasionally occurs as a result of bowel disease and a sigmoidoscopy and barium enema may be necessary, either before or after clearance of the rectum depending upon the practicalities of the situation. A single enema or suppository is extremely unlikely to adequately clear the rectum and descending colon of retained faecal residues. It is necessary to continue to administer intermittent enemas until the rectum can be seen and felt to be clear and the descending colon found to be free of faecal residues on palpation. Occasionally, a plain abdominal film is necessary to confirm this. Having cleared the impaction, the next step is to maintain this state of affairs by keeping the patient's bowel habit regular with the aid of a bran or mild laxative regime. Aggravating factors, such as codeine containing analgesics should also be avoided. Additional fibre in the diet, in the form of bran, is probably best tried initially, in order to avoid the need for laxatives if possible. A useful bran regime is described below:

> Initially, two teaspoonfuls of bran a day are mixed with a semiliquid medium, increasing the dose by the same amount every three or four days (i.e. twice weekly) until the desired effect is obtained. If there has been no results by the time two tablespoons are being consumed each day, it is unlikely to be sufficient on its own, and it may be necessary to add a mild laxative to the regime.

Neurological damage can lead to faecal incontinence in a variety of ways, but

---

Useful advice for old people and their relatives

The prevention of constipation

The daily use of laxatives should be discouraged, although it can be difficult to break a habit which has lasted for decades. An increase in fibre intake should be suggested instead, but they should be told to start with a small amount of fibre, as described in the text, or one slice of wholemeal bread for example, and then increase the amount. A large helping of Allbran or Bran can cause colic and explosive bowel actions in some people.

the commonest is that occurring in a confused or demented patient. If the latter is responsible, it will usually be discovered that the patient is passing formed motions rather than the semiliquid material typical of faecal soiling due to impaction. It is necessary to remember, however, that faecal impaction can occur, and frequently does, in demented patients. If a treatable cause has not been discovered, faecal incontinence is often best treated by using a constipating drug, e.g. codeine phosphate, and arranging for an artificial bowel evacuation twice weekly with the help of an enema. Particular care must be taken with this regime to avoid faecal impaction!

INCONTINENCE OF URINE

The diagnosis and management of incontinence of urine is often a perplexing problem with so many theoretical aspects that on occasions it is difficult to know where to start. In the elderly it is best to adopt a practical step-by-step approach, and the following is a suggested sequence of diagnostic and management steps.

1. Exclude apparent incontinence

By this is meant those circumstances where a patient is, in common parlance, 'caught short'. In reality they do have control of micturition to some extent, but for some reason they are unable to get to the toilet or their bottle quickly enough. Probably one of the commonest examples is the urgency or frequency associated with infection in the lower urinary tract, and not infrequently it may also be the result of urgency caused by a potent diuretic. The loop diuretics, i.e. frusemide and bumetanide, are the commonest causes of the latter. A careful history and examination of a sterile midstream specimen of urine will help indicate whether one of these factors is responsible, or as is occasionally the case, a contributory factor.

Another circumstance in which apparent incontinence arises is the bed-bound patient who uses the bottle, but who manages to spill some of the urine after he has passed it. If this happens at night, the patient's memory of the events occurring in the preceding hours may be somewhat hazy and often they are not certain how they managed to become wet.

Although there are many other situations which may lead to apparent incontinence, there is one other situation which particularly merits attention, and this is the patient who finds himself in unfamiliar surroundings. It is not unusual for a person to become incontinent shortly after admission to an old persons' home for example, when they were previously continent. This is not just caused by the personal upset at being in a different environment, but probably also in many cases because they are unable to orientate themselves and find the toilet quickly enough, or because the toilet is considerably further away from their own room or the day room than it was from their living room or bed at home. In these circumstances it may take a while for the patient to adjust, and if this process is proving traumatic, a bed-side commode or bottle may well overcome the difficulties as far as nocturnal incontinence is concerned. A careful history and an awareness of the different environment into which a patient has moved may well lead to greater understanding of this problem when it arises. A flow-diagram of the management of apparent incontinence is shown in Fig. 3.1.

2. Retention with overflow

This should be excluded next and it is usually not difficult to ascertain. A full bladder can be felt bimanually or percussed and pressure over the lower

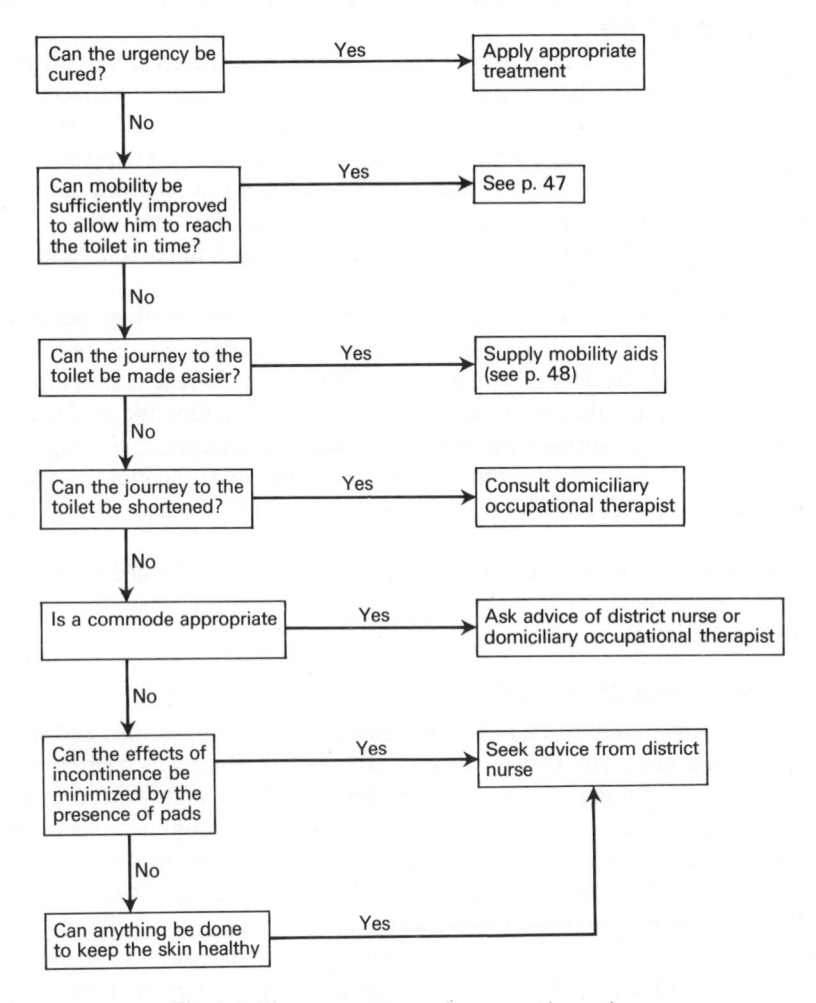

Fig. 3.1. The management of apparent incontinence.

abdomen will often lead to the patient experiencing a feeling of the need to micturate. If necessary, a plain abdominal X-ray will show a large soft tissue mass arising out of the pelvis. If retention of urine is confirmed the first step is to exclude faecal impaction as its cause, and although this is also frequently associated with faecal soiling, this is not always so. The treatment of faecal impaction is considered on page 49. Another common cause of retention with overflow is the prescription of anticholinergic drugs, especially tricyclic antidepressants and antiparkinsonian treatment, as well as di-isopyramide which is currently gaining popularity as an anti-arrhythmic compound. Retention with overflow after the prescription of any of these drugs may act on its own or aggravate a pre-existing condition. The first step therefore is to exclude faecal impaction and the patient's drugs and this is usually simple and does not require hospital referral.

The next commonest cause is probably prostatic hypertrophy if the patient is male, in which case he should be referred to a urologist for further consideration. The diagnosis will require confirmation with an IVP and the bladder may need draining with a catheter as a temporary measure. It is not correct to assume that a patient is too old for surgery, and a TUR especially is a relatively safe and simple procedure even in the disabled. In some patients where this is not appropriate, a catheter draining into a discreetly placed thigh collecting bag may well be the long-term solution to their problems.

In theory, there are many other causes for retention with overflow, but in the elderly they are less common than those mentioned above. Occasionally, an atonic neurogenic bladder occurs as a complication of diabetic neuropathy or tabes dorsalis, when the history and other evidence of autonomic dysfunction or syphilis may indicate such a possibility. In general, however, these diagnoses are best left to the urologist and it is probable that in any patient in whom incontinence is associated with retention of urine, referral for a further opinion is mandatory.

On the practical side, if it is decided to empty a large distended bladder, it must be remembered that this should be done slowly to avoid the risk of intravesical haemorrhage from delicate vesical veins.

3. Stress incontinence and senile vaginitis

There are two conditions that are particularly important in women and merit consideration next. The first of these is stress incontinence which often dates back to pelvic floor damage occurring during child birth, and which may also be associated with a prolapse. The nature of this type of incontinence is usually apparent from the history and examination, and usually requires referral to a gynaecological clinic, although it is often worth trying a pessary first.

Senile vaginitis is associated with incontinence because some of the urethral tissue and the trigone at the base of the bladder have the same embryological origin as the vagina. A local oestrogen preparation, as well as treating the vaginitis, will also often remedy the incontinence. Occasionally oral hormone preparations are necessary, but these are associated with severe side-effects. Whichever regime is adopted intermittent courses are required, the interval between being gauged in each particular patient on a trial and error basis.

4. Mental impairment

Incontinence is often associated with intellectual impairment whether the result of an acute confusional state or part of an existing dementia. When associated with an acute confusional state this is usually obvious and attention to and remedy of the underlying disorder is associated with a return of continence. In more chronic mental impairment, however, the situation is more difficult to resolve and often responds best to regular bladder emptying in conjunction with an incontinence chart, recording frequency and time of the episodes of incontinence. This may help indicate the most appropriate times to toilet a patient, and sometimes results in the establishment of a regular pattern.

It is also important to remember that sedative drugs, both prescribed during the daytime or at night, may also lead to incontinence because of a diminished awareness of the need to void urine. This is most commonly a problem at night when associated with the prescription of hypnotics. In the latter circumstance, discontinuation of the drug or substitution with a short-acting preparation which promotes sleep but does not continue to impair the conscious level may well help rectify the problem.

5. The uninhibited neurogenic bladder

This is unfortunately the situation in many elderly patients, and is often irremediable. Lesions involving the frontal cortex are commonly involved, but damage to the other parts of the cerebrum may also be responsible. The patient is unable to prevent spontaneous bladder contractions, such as those that inform us that our bladder is full and which we constantly override until such time that it is convenient to pass urine. A cystometrogram is required to diagnose this with certainty, and geriatric referral is usually indicated to enable this to be arranged. Some pharmacological agents are occasionally helpful and it is often worth trying preparations such as emepromium bromide and/or flavoxate before resorting to other measures. They need to be taken at an appropriate time in relation to the incontinence and a chart is usually helpful in this respect. Finally, it must be remembered that they have side-effects and also should not be used in patients with glaucoma.

6. Psychological incontinence

Some elderly people are incontinent for psychological reasons of which they are not fully aware. Common examples are:

Punishment incontinence – usually to punish relatives.

Attention-seeking incontinence – consider how much more attention someone in an old people's home receives if he is incontinent, compared with the amount he receives if he takes himself to the toilet in time.

Avoidance incontinence – for example to avoid admission to an old people's home.

It is uncommon for psychological factors to be the sole cause of the incontinence, but they often complicate the problem and influence the severity of it.

Unfortunately, in many patients the incontinence has a multifactorial basis and diagnosis and treatment of one contributory pathology does not always lead to the restitution of continence. On the other hand, incontinence is such a disabling impediment both physically and socially that it is well worth systematically going through all the steps in every incontinent patient.

The management of incontinence

After diagnosis of the cause and treatment, if treatment is possible, the management of incontinence has to be planned with the old person and his relatives.

Objectives of management
1. To protect the dignity of the patient.
2. To protect the skin of the patient.
3. To save the old person, his relatives and helpers from unnecessary work.

The advice of the district nurse is of central importance to the family in achieving these objectives, but referral to hospital may be useful, particularly if the hospital has a specialist incontinence advice service, usually a nurse or physiotherapist, who can try out the full range of aids and appliances. The many aids which are available can be arranged in order of acceptability and effectiveness in preventing damage to the skin. The most acceptable should be tried first.

Incontinence aids in order of acceptability

1. Urinals. Male urinals bottles and female urinals such as the 'St. Peter's boat', or fuba seal urinals are very useful for people whose main problem is mobility.

2. Plastic pants with absorbent pads. A wide range of these are now available.

3. Catheterization. In those patients in whom no treatable cause for the problem is found, the choice of long-term solution is limited. It is easier in men for whom there is a variety of appliances and urinals available. These tend to be less helpful at night, although very satisfactory during the daytime, particularly in someone who has their mental faculties about them. Although Paul's tubing is used in hospital from time to time, there are many practical problems in its usage and it probably is not very helpful in the majority of patients at home. A catheter draining into a discreetly placed thigh collecting bag attached to a waist band is probably the most satisfactory long-term solution for many people.

Nocturnal incontinence

Relatives need information about the prevention of incontinence at night. Firstly they should be told that limitation of fluid in the evening is not effective and that it can cause problems. Secondly, the need for a commode or urinal in the bedroom should be discussed, even when the old person is able to reach the toilet during the day.

The risk of falls at night due to a combination of postural hypotension and peripheral vasodilation can be prevented by leaving a landing light on, and the provision of a commode or urinal.

If nocturnal incontinence is a problem, medication should be reviewed. The half-life of many tranquillizers is increased in old age, and even if the old person is not receiving a hypnotic, the effects of his daytime medication may be contributing to his nocturnal incontinence. If he is receiving a hypnotic this can be withdrawn with the substitute of a more active daily programme and a settled evening activity pattern to establish pre-sleep ritual.

Nocturnal incontinence check-list

1. Is medication a contributory factor?
2. Would a commode or urinal help?
3. Does the old person have enough light to see what he is doing?
4. Have the relatives or the home-help been advised on the best way to make up the old person's bed?

Again the advice of the district nurse is of vital importance.

Incontinence counselling

Although we discuss this topic last it is of primary importance to take into account the emotional aspects of incontinence from the moment of presentation. Incontinence gives rise to feelings of disgust, fear, shame, humiliation, and depression, which may be followed by apathy and hopelessness. For the relatives it can be a source of frustration and anger, 'the last straw'. It is therefore essential that the affected person and his relatives be given the time and the encouragement to discuss their feelings about one of the most feared problems of old age.

Incontinence check-list

1. Is the problem really incontinence with complete loss of control, or is it 'apparent incontinence' due to a combination of urgency and immobility.
2. When apparent incontinence has been excluded, a five-step assessment is indicated:

Management of common problems in the elderly

Step	Possible cause	Test
1	Retention with overflow faecal impaction prostatic hypertrophy	Rectal examination
2	Stress incontinence or senile vaginitis	Vaginal examination at least or inspection while patient performs cough test
3	Mental impairment	Perform simple mental assessment. Review drugs and exclude alcohol abuse
4	Psychological factors	Review social significance of incontinence
5	Neurogenic bladder	Referral for full assessment with cystometrogram

---

Useful advice to old people and their relatives

Controlling the smell

Soak soiled or wet clothes or linen as soon as possible.

Dispose of incontinent pads by wrapping them in newspaper or putting them in plastic bags as soon as possible, then put the 'parcel' in a larger plastic bag.

Try Nilodar which is a neutralizing deodorant to combat smells. It actually neutralizes smells and needs only a few drops in the commode or pad. It is available from most pharmacists.

Try to keep the house and room well ventilated.

Remember that the old person may not detect the smell if he never leaves it.

> **Useful advice to old people and their relatives**
>
> *Coping with the laundry*
>
> The two main difficulties are smell and staining. Both get worse when bedding is exposed to the air. Wet or soiled clothing or bed-linen should be removed as soon as possible and soaked in cold water in a covered bucket. Napisan should be added to the water and the clothing can then be washed in the usual way.
>
> Biological powders are not necessary if soiled clothes and sheets are soaked quickly.
>
> Enquiry should be made about the possibility of help with laundry from Incontinence Laundry Service.

JAUNDICE

Jaundice is investigated along similar lines to those used in younger patients, but the results may be more difficult to interpret as other diseases may also be reflected in the biochemical findings, e.g. bone disease causing an elevation of the alkaline phosphatase. Since it is difficult to estimate the different isoenzymes of alkaline phosphatase it is usual to check a 5-nucleotidase level whenever there is any doubt since this is only raised when there is liver disease and is unaffected by conditions of bone. The history and examination are often revealing when determining the most likely cause for a patient's jaundice, for instance, signs of chronic liver disease indicate long-standing hepatic damage rather than a more acute episode, such as a stone blocking the common bile-duct. The normal range of bilirubin level should be taken as the same in older patients as in younger people.

Jaundice is most conveniently divided into the usual three major types, i.e. obstructive jaundice and hepatocellular jaundice which occur more commonly than haemolytic jaundice.

Obstructive jaundice

Obstructive jaundice is probably the commonest form of jaundice in the elderly and is characterized by finding an elevated alkaline phosphatase. Although the transaminases are also usually raised, relatively speaking this is to a lesser degree than the alkaline phosphatase. Although rarely tested for there will also be the usual findings in the urine (see below) in conjunction with the history of dark urine and pale stools. It is not uncommon for a gall-stone to produce a severe jaundice and yet itself be painless, even though the old adage that painless obstructive jaundice is due to a neoplasm is very often true.

Amongst the commonest neoplasms are those of the head of the pancreas, the stomach, multiple secondaries from other sites, and very rarely a carcinoma of the biliary tract itself. If a more diffuse condition, such as a lymphoma, is responsible there will usually be splenic enlargement and possibly lympthadenopathy.

Drugs do not cause jaundice in the elderly as frequently as they once did since phenothiazines, especially chlorpromazine, are not prescribed as often as they once were. Nevertheless, they should be considered as a potential cause and as well as phenothiazines, sulphonylureas, and erythromycin are amongst the drugs that can be responsible.

Most patients with obstructive jaundice should be admitted to hospital, but if the jaundice is not severe and the patient is well enough, it may be possible to arrange further investigations as an outpatient. Occasionally a plain abdominal film will reveal gall-stones. The majority of these, however, are radiolucent and even when found they are not necessarily responsible for the jaundice, being an incidental finding. Particularly helpful are a liver scan or an ultrasound and it is sometimes possible to arrange for one of these to be performed urgently to confirm the diagnosis. This can be a help in deciding whether or not the patient should be admitted to hospital, and will also show secondary deposits if present, allowing some patients the possibility of terminal care at home. An oral cholecystogram is unhelpful if the patient is clinically jaundiced, but intravenous cholangiography may reveal useful information if the bilirubin level is less than 35 mmol/l (2 mg per 100 ml). Sometimes barium contrast studies are appropriate and may show the presence of an upper GI tract tumour.

Hepatocellular jaundice

In hepatocellular jaundice the SGOT and LDH levels rise, relatively speaking, to a higher level than the alkaline phosphatase. The urinary abnormalities are described below. The commonest cause of hepatocellular jaundice in the elderly is probably alcoholic cirrhosis. This may well be suspected from the history, although alcoholics are extremely adept at minimizing or denying their alcohol intake, but there will usually be evidence of long-standing liver disease on physical examination, including signs of portal hypertension. A barium swallow will often show the presence of oesophageal varices.

Haemolytic jaundice

This is an uncommon finding in older people and is most easily confirmed in the general practice setting by testing the urine (see below). A mild degree of haemolysis, however, may be present in untreated pernicious anaemia because of the shortened life-span of the macrocytic red cells. Other causes of severe haemolysis which should be suspected in the elderly include a severe infection, usually with septicaemia, and pulmonary infarction in a patient who has congestive cardiac failure. It can also be caused by certain drugs and amongst those that should be suspected are methyldopa, mefenamic acid, penicillin, phenacetin, and salicylates.

Old people rarely suffer with hereditary spherocytosis and paroxysmal nocturnal haemoglobinuria, but idiopathic autoimmune haemolytic anaemias may occur at any age and may be associated with warm or cold antibodies. The cold antibody variety is more prevalent in the elderly and is often associated with Raynaud's phenomenon and haemoglobinuria in addition to the anaemia. A positive direct Coombs' test and an excess of cold antibodies in the serum confirm the diagnosis.

Other causes of haemolytic anaemia in the elderly include the secondary autoimmune disorders, which are often associated with other underlying conditions, in particular lymphomas, paraproteinaemias, and collagenoses. A patient with a haemolytic anaemia is probably best admitted to hospital, although the treatment of the anaemia itself may be relatively simple if it is due to one of the warm antibody types, since steroids are often helpful as maybe immunosupressive therapy, although it may be necessary to resort to splenectomy in some cases. These measures are occasionally beneficial in the cold antibody types, but these are more difficult to treat.

Enzyme abnormalities

Alkaline phosphatase

The normal range for alkaline phosphatase levels is probably the same in older as in younger patients. The two most important sources of this enzyme are liver and bone. Most of the hepatic alkaline phosphatase is concentrated in the epithelium of the bile-ducts, which probably explains the high levels obtained in an obstructive process. The highest levels of alkaline phosphatase may be associated with a tumour of the biliary duct epithelium, although this is uncommon.

Osteolytic abnormalities of bone require an accompanying osteoblastic reaction for there to be an elevation of the alkaline phosphatase. Most commonly this is associated with secondary bone tumours, in particular from the breast and prostate. Occasionally, it also happens in multiple myeloma. In all of these conditions, however, the alkaline phosphatase may also be elevated because of hepatic involvement. Two other bony causes of an elevated alkaline phosphatase are Paget's disease and the presence of a healing fracture.

A routine biochemical screen usually includes liver function tests and bone biochemistry and will therefore in the majority of cases help to differentiate between a hepatic and bony cause for the elevated alkaline phosphatase level. If, however, the calcium, phosphate, and liver function tests are normal, it may be necessary to estimate the 5-nucleotidase level. This is an enzyme that is specific to liver disease and indicates that the alkaline phosphatase is raised because of hepatic impairment, although occasionally there may be coincidental bone involvement, e.g. with secondary deposits in both sites.

Lactate dehydrogenase (LDH)

An elevated LDH may be an accompaniment of many conditions. Most commonly it indicates hepatic impairment or a recent myocardial infarction. In the latter case there is the typical pattern of a peak approximately three to four days after the infarction has occurred. It may also rise in pulmonary infarction, in association with a megaloblastic anaemia and occasionally in a patient with a cerebrovascular accident. The underlying aetiology can be ascertained with the help of a biochemical screen, a blood count, and an ECG.

Aspartase transaminase (SGOT)

This is usually elevated in liver disease and high levels are a marker of hepatocellular pathology, since the rise in obstructive jaundice is usually moderate. It also rises after a myocardial infarction with peak values a little in advance of the peak in the LDH level.

Biliary pigments in the urine (Table 3.1)

Bilirubin

Bilirubin in the urine indicates the presence of obstructive jaundice. The obstruction to the outflow of bile results in spill over into the blood of some conjugated bilirubin which is secreted in the urine and conversely, the absence of bile in the bowel produces the pale stools and loss of urobilinogen from the urine. The presence of the latter relies upon the absorption from the bowel and excretion by the kidney.

Table 3.1. *Biliary pigments in the urine*

	Bilirubin	Urobilinogen
Normal	none	small amount
Prehepatic jaundice	none	increased
Hepatocellular jaundice	present	may be increased then absent, depending on cause
Posthepatic jaundice (obstruction)	present	absent

Urobilinogen

Urobilinogen in excess in the urine is usually a consequence of a haemolytic process. A haemolytic anaemia is best confirmed with the aid of a blood count and film, and a Coombs' test, which will be positive in the majority of the autoimmune haemolytic anaemias. Initially these should be considered to be drug induced until proved otherwise as described above. Occasionally, a haemolytic process can be complicated by an obstructive element owing to the formation of pigment gall stones, and this situation may be difficult to unravel.

Treatment

Unless the cause of the jaundice is immediately apparent and does not require onward referral, or the disease is static, most jaundiced patients should probably be referred to hospital. It is particularly important to exclude remediable conditions and also those that can be ameliorated. Examples of these include the silent stone and the bypass procedure in somebody with malignancy at the head of the pancreas. In the former case, the patient can look forward to a normal life-span after a successful operation, and in the latter often several months of symptom-free life until terminal care is required.

LEG ULCERS

There are many potential causes of leg ulcers, varying from the commonly encountered arterial insufficiency and ulceration associated with varicose veins, to less common conditions such as those associated with severe ulcerative colitis and the haemolytic anaemias. It is important to try and establish the cause wherever possible since the treatment for one condition may aggravate another if the diagnosis is in error, e.g. elevation of the legs for stasis ulceration in a patient with vascular insufficiency. There may be indications in the history which will lead one to suspect the presence of a particular type of ulceration, for instance diabetes mellitus indicating the possibility of peripheral vascular disease.

Varicose ulcers can usually be suspected from their characteristic site, the associated pigmentation, and the history of varicose veins. The presence of oedema may also be a helpful factor in arriving at the diagnosis, but it is more difficult to interpret since there are so many causes of ankle swelling in the elderly. Varicose ulcers are best treated by rest with the legs elevated. Elevating the foot of the bed at night in a patient with no contra-indication (e.g. orthopnea, hiatus hernia, or peripheral vascular disease) will also help speed healing.

Ulcers resulting from peripheral vascular disease are the most difficult to heal. Often all one can do is combine an attempt to promote healing with measures to treat the underlying predisposition, if any, to vascular disease in the hope of slowing down a tendency to ulceration in the future.

In diabetes mellitus the skin may break down just because of vascular insufficiency, but also because of the neurological sequelae of this condition, which results in impaired awareness of local trauma.

Any patient in whom there is ankle oedema and who sustains minor trauma is a candidate for a wound that will be slow to heal. It is as important to treat the underlying oedema as the wound itself and this will require tubigrip type stockingette rather than diuretic therapy unless the oedema is caused by cardiac failure.

In bed-bound patients pressure sores are also a cause of leg ulceration, but these are discussed elsewhere (p. 71).

The initial treatment of a leg ulcer consists in looking for and remedying where possible any underlying cause, as mentioned earlier, cleaning the ulcer with either hydrogen peroxide or half-strength Eusol solution, and applying simple dressings. Chronic leg ulcers often support a variety of bacteria, whose importance is a matter of controversy. If there is evidence of surrounding cellulitis to a significant extent, systemic antibiotic therapy rather than topical application is indicated. Topical antibiotics may do more harm than good and often precipitate contact dermatitis with an aggravation of the ulceration. It is considered by some authorities that anaerobic organisms, especially streptococci and bacteroides species may play a more significant role than formerly recognized. A seven-day course of metronidazole (e.g. 400 mg t.d.s) may speed healing if an anaerobic infection is discovered.

A patient's nutritional state may also be important in promoting healing, and if there is any cause to suspect malnutrition, attention should be paid to the patient's diet and the possible need for vitamin replacement.

Recalcitrant leg ulcers are probably best referred to hospital for further consideration, which may involve skin biopsy and/or the possibility of grafting in appropriate cases, although many ulcers will heal with a spell of bed-rest and intensive nursing support.

MALABSORPTION

Malabsorption is indicated by finding a similar biochemical and haematological picture to that described under the heading of malnutrition (see below). The absence of steatorrhoea does not exclude this condition and many elderly people have significant malabsorption without any evidence of steatorrhoea at all. If malabsorption is suspected, barium studies of the stomach and small bowel are required and these can be organized from general practice, as also can a faecal fat estimation if the patient is co-operative. If a jejunal biopsy is necessary, however, this is best undertaken in a hospital setting, even if only as a day case.

In many elderly people malasorption is a consequence of a previous partial gastrectomy and associated blind-loop syndrome, but it may also be caused by one of the chronic diarrhoeas, such as Crohn's disease or small bowel diverticula.

It must not be forgotten, and should be considered before embarking upon additional investigations, that malabsorption can occur as a result of the medications a patient is taking. Drugs that are sometimes involved include Neomycin and other broad-spectrum antibiotics, some purgatives, e.g. phenolphthalein, and para-aminosalicylic acid (PAS). There are also of course other conditions, such as long-standing congestive cardiac failure and coeliac disease, although the latter is rarely diagnosed for the first time in old age.

Treatment is centred around correcting the underlying abnormality and replacing the nutritional deficiencies. In many instances, it is impossible for this to be organized without further referral. If no cause is found, however, a second opinion is probably necessary.

MALNUTRITION

The Department of Health and Social Security carried out a nutritional survey of old people at home, following a cohort of 483 people aged over 70, over a five-year period. As with other diseases the prevalence of malnutrition rose with age and 12 per cent of the men and 8 per cent of the women were malnourished.

The survey revealed two sets of results that are helpful to the person trying to assess the nutritional status of an old person in his own home. The first was that malnutrition was associated with certain medical and social conditions and that these could be regarded as risk factors for malnutrition. If one or more is present, malnutrition should be suspected and excluded (Table 3.2).

Table 3.2. *Medical and social conditions associated with malnutrition*

Condition	Special feature of malnutrition associated with condition, in addition to generalized malnutrition
Partial gastrectomy	Nutritional anaemia
Chronic bronchitis and emphysema	
Confusion	
Depression	
Edentulous and failure to use dentures	Fibre deficiency, constipation and incontinence
Difficulty in swallowing	
Housebound	Vitamin D deficiency
No regular cooked meals	
In social class IV or V	
In receipt of supplementary benefit	

The second set of findings which were helpful was the distinction between physical signs which were associated with malnutrition to a statistically signifcant degree from those which were not.

Physical signs significantly associated with malnutrition

Wasted appearance.
Sublingual haemorrhages.
Sublingual varicosities.
Red seborrheic nasolabial folds.
Hyperkeratosis.
Inappropriate pigmentation of exposed skin.

In this study a smooth atrophic tongue, flat nails and koilonychia, angular stomatitis, and cheilosis were not associated with malnutrition.

It is often difficult to confirm a history of dietary inadequacy from the person themselves and it may be necessary to seek confirmation from a reliable third party. Examination will often indicate the consequences of nutritional deficiencies, such as the classical changes of iron deficiency and an anaemia, and the signs of vitamin B_{12} deficiency. There will also be biochemical evidence and it is not uncommon to find a low serum albumin, signs of osteomalacia, i.e. a low calcium, and an elevated alkaline phosphatase. A routine blood count will also show evidence of an anaemia which is usually hypochromic and microcytic. If these abnormalities are present, but the dietary intake appears to be adequate then it is necessary to consider the possibility of malabsorption as described in more detail below.

This problem is remedied by prescribing the appropriate vitamin supplements, considering the necessity for meals on wheels or attendance at a lunch club, and referring the problem to the Social Worker and relatives so that the underlying difficulties which have led to a deficient diet can be tackled. If the weight loss or biochemical abnormalities continue, it is probable that there is another factor involved and referral for further investigation is necessary.

Dental problems

One of the reasons why some older people do not eat enough is that they have difficulty with eating meat, vegetables, and foods with a high content of cereal fibre, either because their teeth or gums are painful, or because their dentures are ill fitting and cause them pain. Like younger people, old people should consult a dentist regularly whether or not they have symptoms, and they should also seek help promptly when they develop symptoms. Those with teeth should see their dentist at least once a year. Those who have dentures should consult a dentist every second year, provided that they do not develop symptoms in between these check-ups. Unfortunately many old people do not see a dentist as often as this for three reasons:

1. The low expectations of older people, their relatives and professional people.
2. Their immobility (see p. 45).
3. The increasing difficulty in which people have finding a dentist willing to treat them 'on the NHS'.

If a personal approach to a friend who is a dentist is of no avail, it is worthwhile seeking the advice of the District Dental Officer, and it may be worthwhile asking whether an old person could be seen by the dentist who visits the day hospital, even if he has no medical need for day hospital attendance.

Useful advice for old people and their relatives

Paying for dental care

Old people who receive supplementary pension or have a low income receive free dental treatment and dentures. The dentist has copies of Form F1D, but it is essential to ensure that the dentist is willing to give treatment on the National Health Service before each course of treatment: no help can be given towards private fees.

MYOCARDIAL INFARCTION

The treatment of myocardial infarction in the elderly is similar to that in younger patients. There are, however, one or two specific issues that are worth mentioning, and these are summarized below.

The need to admit to hospital

It is now generally accepted that many patients, especially the elderly, with a myocardial infarction do not require hospital treatment. Many elderly patients in particular do not wish to be sent to hospital, and in an uncomplicated myocardial infarction it is very reasonable to treat the patient at home. A patient who is shocked, however, who develops an arrhythmia, or who is found to be in heart failure should be admitted to hospital as soon as possible. It will also be necessary to admit any patient who lives on their own, or otherwise has nobody to care for them.

Analgesics

Many of our elders develop myocardial infarction without pain, and if present it is often not very severe. Diamorphine with an anti-emetic may be necessary, but it is often possible to prescribe a milder preparation. Whatever the circumstances prompt pain relief is extremely important.

Bed-rest

Mobilization of an elderly patient following a myocardial infarction is usually started the day after the infarction as long as there are no complications and the patient is pain free. Initially this takes place slowly and gradually increasing over a period of a week to ten days. The reappearance or persistence of pain, or the development of heart failure or an arrhythmia indicates the need to return the patient to bed, even though there is a risk of developing a DVT and the other consequences of bed-rest in the elderly.

If it is necessary to treat cardiac failure or a dysrrhythmia at home, a standard therapeutic approach should be used. It must be remembered though that small doses of the drug should be tried initially, and that a loop-diuretic (i.e Frusemide or Bumetanide) should only be used to promote an urgent diuresis. If the patient's recovery does not prove to be as straightforward as originally anticipated, referral to hospital is usually necessary.

OEDEMA OF THE ANKLES

Most people who present with ankle oedema are unlikely to require diuretics. One should not assume that it is a symptom of cardiac failure unless there is other clinical evidence to support this, e.g. an elevated JVP, bilateral basal crepitations, or a third heart sound. If it is in fact due to heart failure, as well as treating this it is important to look for any underlying cause for the onset of the cardiac failure since occasionally a treatable condition will be discovered. Although ischaemic heart disease is by far the commonest cause, hypertension, valvular heart disease, anaemia, and thyrotoxicosis not infrequently cause cardiac failure in the elderly.

Other causes of ankle oedema include the following.

1. Immobility – although this may be unilateral, e.g. after a cerebrovascular accident, when it may be aggravated by diminished venous tone, or a DVT, oedema due to generalized immobility is more frequently bilateral and is due to a combination of the effects of gravity and the lack of muscle pump action.

2. Hypoproteinaemia – this essentially means a low serum albumin for which there are many potential causes. These include liver disease, inadequate nutrition, malabsorption, and less commonly the nephrotic syndrome.

3. Drugs – amongst those pharmaceutical preparations which cause fluid retention, the most commonly used include steroids (especially corticosteroids and stilboestrol), carbenoxolone sodium, and non-steroidal anti-inflammatory drugs such as phenylbutazone.

4. Venous obstruction – thrombosis in the deep veins of the legs occurs far more commonly than is suspected and should be carefully watched for after a cerebrovascular accident, a coronary thrombosis, and in people with neoplastic disease. Deep venous thromboses are also a post-operative hazard in people who have recently undergone surgery, and with the trend towards ever earlier discharge home post-operatively for many procedures, this has to be borne in mind. Typically unilaterally, they can of course occur bilaterally, although bilateral ankle oedema is more commonly secondary to venous obstruction in the pelvic veins or inferior vena cava. The latter may be precipitated not only by an abdominal mass, but also by ascites.

Varicose veins are also associated with ankle oedema in some patients, and in these cases it is the increase in pressure in the column of blood in the vessels rather than thrombosis that is responsible.

5. Lymphatic obstruction – this most commonly arises as a result of neoplastic deposits in lymph nodes. It is then often unilateral.

Occasionally, one comes across a patient with Milroy's disease in which there is a congenital absence of lymphatics, but they will have had swollen legs for most of their life and are unlikely to present with it as a problem for the first time in old age.

It is also important not to forget that the constrictive effects of some clothes can result in venous stasis and an aggravation of ankle oedema. An example of this is the elasticated legging of old ladies underwear, and the practice often employed of keeping stockings in position by twisting their tops. These are not always obvious after the patient has been undressed by a nurse ready for examination. They are rarely, however, responsible for more than a little fluid accumulation.

Investigation

The cause of ankle oedema is usually apparent from a careful history and examination supported by a full blood count, and estimation of urea and electrolytes together with a biochemical screen. If a more serious condition is suspected, or a DVT, referral to hospital is necessary, but in many cases treatment can be instituted without further investigation.

Management

1. The first step of course is to treat any underlying condition if this is possible.
2. The next practical step is to elevate the foot of the bed at night in order to re-distribute the oedema. This is not appropriate, however, if the patient is suffering with cardiac failure because of the risk of orthopnea, oesophageal reflux secondary to a hiatus hernia, or in someone with peripheral arterial disease.
3. Elevation of the feet during the daytime should also be advocated, but is usually unsatisfactory because the patients find it rather uncomfortable.
4. Supportive treatment. Crepe bandages are unsatisfactory in the elderly in many cases because they can be very difficult for an old person to put on properly. Elastic stockings are often advocated, but they too can be a struggle to wear, and in many cases tubigrip type stockingette will suffice. Exercising ankles and knees may help.

OSTEOMALACIA

Osteomalacia differs from osteoporosis because of a deficiency of calcification of the normal bone matrix or osteoid. It is most commonly caused by vitamin D deficiency of a dietary origin, or in consequence of malabsorption. In some cases, especially in immigrant populations, it has been described in relation to lack of exposure to sunlight, and may also be a feature of renal disease since vitamin D metabolism is impaired in the presence of chronic renal failure. Certain drugs, especially anticonvulsants, also interfere with vitamin D metabolism in the liver and can precipitate osteomalacia.

Presentation

The presenting features may be non-specific in nature and consist of vague reports of weakness and aches and pains. These should be taken seriously especially if they are accompanied by difficulty in performing normal daily activities such as climbing stairs. Osteomalacia is characterized by proximal muscle weakness as well as the skeletal deformities resulting from softening of the bones themselves, resulting in features such as the kyphosis so often seen.

Investigations

An X-ray is often extremely helpful in confirming the diagnosis since not only will it reveal generalized decalcification, but possibly also the pseudofractures known as Looser's zones which are areas of decalcification presenting as apparent cracks in the cortex and best seen in the axillary border of the scapula, the femoral neck and the upper end of the humerus amongst other sites. This finding is diagnostic.

Biochemical abnormalities include a raised alkaline phosphatase, a calcium that is often low, but may be normal, and a low phosphate. The calcium and phosphate levels respond rapidly to treatment even if this consists only of a hospital diet with an adequate vitamin D intake. Diagnosis can therefore be difficult on occasion unless Looser's zones are found on the X-ray, or a bone biopsy is performed.

Treatment

This is oral or intramuscular vitamin D in the standard doses. Calcium supplements are also required in many cases. All patients on vitamin D and/or calcium should have their renal function and plasma calcium levels monitored regularly.

An underlying cause should be sought and where appropriate treated. If this can be remedied long-term vitamin and calcium supplements may be avoided, although initially necessary. Though the calcium and phosphate levels may return to normal rapidly, the alkaline phosphatase will take much longer to return to normal.

OSTEOPOROSIS

Osteoporosis is caused by a loss of bone substance, i.e. both protein, matrix, and calcium salts, the substance left being fully mineralized unless there is concurrent osteomalacia, which not infrequently occurs in older patients. Its presence should be suspected when the typical symptoms present in any patient with a predisposing medical history including Cushing's disease and steroid therapy, rheumatoid arthritis, and immobilization. Perhaps the commonest presenting symptom is of back pain associated with a collapsed vertebral body, or fracture of a bone elsewhere such as the femoral neck and a Colles' fracture of the wrist.

For practical purposes the diagnosis can be made radiologically, but where there is doubt, e.g. where it may have important consequences on the further management of a patient on steroids, or the possibility of concurrent osteomalacia exists, hospital referral for bone biopsy is usually necessary. In pure osteoporosis there are no abnormalities in the plasma calcium, phosphate, and alkaline phosphatase.

Treatment is controversial, probably ineffective, and as usual preventive measures are best, although this is not always possible. Anabolic steroids, calcium supplements, and vitamin D analogues have all been advocated, but the best treatment is still a matter of debate. It has been confused because of the tendency in so many elderly people for there to be concurrent osteomalacia, which may not have been apparent in some of the trials of treatment that have been undertaken.

PAGET'S DISEASE OF BONE

The majority of cases of Paget's disease need no treatment or further consideration. It usually affects one or occasionally two or three bones in a particular patient, and most patients remain symptomless. Occasionally problems such as deafness, headaches, and bone pain arise and even the need to purchase a larger size hat if the disease is localized to the skull. Complications include pathological fractures and rarely, but significantly, sarcomatous change. High-output cardiac failure and compression of the spinal cord can occur, but are only seen infrequently. The finding of Paget's disease as an incidental abnormality on an X-ray in a symptomless patient is probably best ignored, but the diagnosis noted in case relevant symptoms emerge at a later date.

Investigation

It is characterized by normal calcium and phosphate levels unless the patient is immobile when the calcium may rise. The alkaline phosphatase is usually elevated, often to quite high levels when the disease is active and it is occasionally diagnosed in this way, i.e. investigation of an incidental finding of a high alkaline phosphatase on a biochemical screen.

Treatment

Initially this is symptomatic and simple analgesics are probably best for pain and discomfort. Calcitonin is also used for pain that does not respond to simple analgesics and when some of the neurological complications ensue, but it has to be given intramuscularly for several months and is probably best initially supervised via a hospital outpatient clinic.

PARKINSONISM

The classical features of parkinsonism are too well known to merit detailed consideration here, but it is important to emphasize the effects of the bradykinesia. This can lead to great difficulty in rising from a chair or getting out of bed, which is often misinterpreted as laziness or awkwardness by others when they see the patient walking on another occasion. This point needs explaining to relatives so that the patient is not unnecessarily maligned. The first and probably most important step when considering parkinsonism in the elderly is to eliminate the side-effects of phenothiazine or related drugs as its cause. It is extremely common, both in hospital and outside, to discover patients taking a drug which induces extrapyramidal side-effects and an antiparkinsonian agent concurrently to counteract these effects, without the relationship between the two being appreciated by the doctor responsible. In the majority of instances the drugs involved can easily be discontinued or reduced in dosage to obviate the need for antiparkinsonian therapy, which in its turn introduces additional and often very disabling side-effects of its own. In addition in many such instances the symptoms are being treated with an l-dopa preparation, which is clearly inappropriate when the rigidity and other signs are phenothiazine induced, since these drugs produce parkinsonism by blocking the receptor sites for dopamine within the basal ganglia. Prescribing an L-dopa combination preparation in an attempt to increase the concentration of dopamine at the appropriate sites does not often significantly improve matters. If it is impossible to withdraw the offending drug completely or reduce its dosage sufficiently to make antiparkinsonian treatment unnecessary, one of the anticholinergic preparations should be prescribed, e.g. Benzhexol or Orphenadrine.

The L-dopa combination preparations, usually L-dopa and carbidopa or L-dopa and benserazide are probably the most effective drugs in the elderly for the treatment of Parkinson's disease. They are more effective in controlling the bradykinesia and rigidity than in relieving the tremor. Since dopamine is an active transmitter at other sites within and outside the brain, side-effects are common particularly with larger doses. For this reason it is important to start with the smallest possible dose and slowly work up taking care to watch out for the onset of gastro-intestinal upset, depression, hallucinations, and confusional states. It is also necessary in people on L-dopa preparations to watch out for the development of the 'on-off effect' which occurs in a small number of patients after long-term treatment. This is marked by rapid intermittent dyskinesia.

The other major group of drugs used in the treatment of parkinsonism are the anticholinergic compounds which have been in use for over a century. Amongst this group are benzhexol which is extremely effective but produces confusion in a large number of elderly patients, and orphenadrine. Other side-effects include postural hypotension, and the aggravation of any tendency towards glaucoma, or retention of urine in men with prostatic hypertrophy.

Amantadine is rarely used in the treatment of Parkinson's disease, or parkinsonism in the elderly, but is worth considering when the other preparations have to be discontinued. It is generally better tolerated, but unfortunately is not so effective. Amongst its side-effects are confusion and fluid retention.

In some patients a combination of drugs is helpful, for example the patient whose salivation may be controlled with a small dose of an anticholinergic agent while an L-dopa preparation is used as the major therapeutic agent. It is also worth adding small doses of anticholinergic drugs to a patient in whom L-dopa preparations have not produced the satisfactory result.

POLYMYALGIA RHEUMATICA

As mentioned elsewhere this is part of the spectrum of disease which includes temporal arteritis. In fact in many patients with symptoms attributable to polymyalgia rheumatica there will be evidence of an arteritis affecting the same sites as in temporal arteritis. The major presenting feature of polymyalgia rheumatica is of pain and stiffness in the proximal limb muscles and the shoulder and pelvic girdles. This is usually worst in the mornings, and generalized constitutional upset including a pyrexia are usually present. It is accompanied by a high ESR and should be treated in the same way as temporal arteritis. The symptoms usually respond dramatically to the steroids, prescription of which is often a useful therapeutic test.

PRESSURE SORES

This is the current name for bed sores. Many people still use the latter term which is often manifestly incorrect. Most people are familiar with the risk of developing pressure sores in the sacral area, over the greater trochanter and over the heels. It is often forgotten, however, that underlying conditions may aggravate a tendency to pressure sores and should be sought in any patient in whom there is a likelihood of these developing. Their presence not only alerts one to the increased risk of a particular patient developing an area of breakdown, but since some of them are amenable to treatment, identification may be helpful in reducing the risk of a sore occurring, or possibly limiting its severity. These factors include hypotension and peripheral vascular disease, as well as malnutrition, anaemia, and urinary or faecal incontinence. Apart from these additional risk factors, pressure sores are particularly likely to arise in any patient who is immobile for any length of time.

Treatment

Any predisposing factor or underlying condition should obviously be treated if this is possible. Catheterization may also help if it is considered that urinary incontinence is aggravating the situation. The main-stay of treatment, however, is regular turning, preferably every two hours, and for this reason a patient in whom pressure sores have arisen may well have to be admitted to hospital. Sheepskin heel pads, ripple mattresses, sorbo rubber rings, and other similar aids are useful agents to prevention but come second best to regular turning and keeping the patient off his pressure area where healing is concerned.

The role of infection is often misunderstood and since it is usually superficial is probably best treated with local antiseptic measures rather than systemic or local antibiotics. Suitable solutions include half-strength Eusol and hydrogen peroxide. If there is severe local cellulitis involving deeper tissues, systemic antibiotics are probably necessary, but a swab should be taken first to indicate which is the most appropriate antibiotic.

72 Management of common problems in the elderly

If there is dead or necrotic tissue in the centre of the sore, this must be removed before there is any chance of the wound healing. Again this is probably easier in hospital, but could easily be undertaken in a community or cottage hospital rather than a district general hospital or a geriatric unit. If a sore takes a long time to heal an opinion from a plastic surgeon is often worthwhile, and it is important to remember if the breakdown has occurred over a bony prominence that there may be infection in the underlying bone. This will usually become apparent radiologically.

Many different agents have been advocated to enhance healing, including maggots, insulin and egg white, oxygen, and sugar, but these probably play only a secondary part if any. Regular turning and keeping the patient off the pressure area being the main-stay of treatment. Ultraviolet light is probably one exception to this and is occasionally helpful in promoting granulation tissue and possibly retarding bacterial overgrowth.

Other measures, especially attention to a patient's state of nutrition, preparations containing streptokinase and similar enzymes, and other preparations marketed for local application are occasionally helpful. They are too numerous to mention in detail, but a similar approach to that mentioned in the discussion of leg ulcers may be helpful (p. 61).

RENAL IMPAIRMENT

Elevation of blood urea

Many elderly people have a blood urea level that is within the normal limits for younger people, i.e. less than 7 mmol/l. Not infrequently, however, it is found to be as high as 10 mmol/l without any evidence of a significant underlying pathology. It is not unreasonable to accept this as normal, but a level greater than 10 always requires further consideration. It is probably best to exclude dehydration in the first instance which will usually be clinically obvious. Dryness of the mouth, tachycardia, reduced skin turgor, and diminished urinary output all indicate dehydration, especially if there is an elevated specific gravity in the urine. The serum creatinine level may also be proportionately lower than the urea, but in the elderly the creatinine can rise as a direct result of dehydration, although this is generally not appreciated. The presence of dehydration can also be surmized by finding an elevated haematocrit and raised serum protein level. The commonest causes include diuretic treatment and pyrexial illness, although any elderly person taking to their bed may reduce their fluid intake.

An increase in protein breakdown, as may occur for instance after an upper gastro-intestinal haemorrhage, can also elevate the blood urea, but this is usually a short-term phenomenon. There is in any case usually supportive evidence indicating that bleeding has occurred. More commonly however increased protein breakdown is a non-specific phenomenon occurring in many illnesses and can also be associated with the use of some drugs, for instance steroids and tetracycline derivatives, as well as being an accompaniment of many fevers. If either of these two conditions, i.e. dehydration or increased protein breakdown, is considered to be the cause of the elevated urea then a repeat estimation when the underlying condition has been corrected should confirm that further investigation is unnecessary.

Chronic renal failure

In chronic renal failure there will be an elevated serum phosphate and uric acid, and a low serum calcium. The patient will usually be acidotic with a low serum bicarbonate, and the potassium may rise. A normochromic anaemia is usually present, often falling to as low as 7 or 8 g per cent. It is surprising how quickly a low haemoglobin can be produced in renal disease, however, and such a low level does not necessarily imply that the duration of the renal failure should be measured in months since it could well be weeks. Detecting protein in the urine will also indicate the presence of kidney damage. If chronic renal failure is suspected it is extremely important to look for any treatable underlying aetiological factors, including a high blood pressure and diabetes mellitus since controlling both of these conditions may well delay further deterioration in renal function. There are other conditions that need excluding and these include prostatic hypertrophy, or obstruction due to stones or more rarely urethral valves. There are of course many chronic conditions for which there is little available treatment and these include chronic pyleonephritis, nephrosclerosis, and diabetic nephropathy.

In addition to the investigations mentioned above it is important to arrange the examination of a fresh specimen of urine. Occasionally, a sterile pyuria is discovered and although this in theory indicates the possibility of renal tract tuberculosis it is not uncommonly due to a partially treated lower urinary tract infection. An IVP is also necessary even if a high-dose infusion method has to be employed, and if this is not easily available in general practice, hospital referral for further investigation at this point is probably indicated. A patient with chronic renal failure referred to a hospital clinic for further investigation will usually be screened for myeloma and collagenoses, as treatment of these conditions is usually worthwhile. There is, however, no reason why all these investigations should not be carried out from the general practice setting.

Amyloid is an uncommon cause of chronic renal failure in the elderly, but is more likely to occur in an older person than in the younger patient. It should be suspected if the renal failure is accompanied by normal sized or slightly enlarged kidneys.

Treatment of chronic renal failure is probably best carried out in the hospital environment, although this does not necessarily need district general hospital facilities. There is little difference between the treatment in younger and older patients, the principles being the same, i.e. controlling fluid and electrolyte balance, correcting the acidosis and restricting protein intake. It is necessary to avoid infection and dehydration if at all possible, but a high index of suspicion should be maintained for both of these conditions since early detection and treatment will often avoid or limit a further reduction in renal function.

Acute renal failure

Acute renal failure in older people is usually of the acute or chronic type. This is indicated by finding the characteristic biochemical and haematological abnormalities already described. Admission to hospital is necessary if it is decided that the condition ought to be treated rather than be allowed to run its natural course in a patient where this is appropriate. The principles of treatment include controlling fluid and electrolyte balance, a high-calorie low-protein diet, vitamin supplements, and sometimes anabolic steroids. If a decision is made to try to treat the patient outside the context of a district general hospital, in addition to the points already mentioned it is particularly important to avoid over-hydration which can result in cardiac failure. Although a severe anaemia should be corrected it must be remembered that there is a high potassium and protein content in stored blood. A patient with moderate anaemia is probably best left untransfused. The other pit-falls to avoid are those of infection, dehydration, and urinary tract obstruction just as in the case of chronic renal failure.

Diagnosis of the underlying pathology is probably most efficiently made in the hospital environment. Since some of the causes of acute renal failure are eminently treatable it is important that this is taken into account when a decision is made about the patient's management.

Associated abnormalities in the urine

Proteinuria

Occasionally proteinuria is caused by contamination, for instance by vaginal secretions in women. Unless there is other frank evidence of renal tract disease, it is important to exclude contamination as a cause of proteinuria before investigating the condition further. Microscopy may reveal vaginal cells confirming contamination from this source. It may also be excluded by carefully repeating the test taking as great care as possible to avoid contamination, although this can be difficult in elderly women.

The commonest cause of proteinuria is probably a lower urinary tract infection. The accompanying bacterial growth and the presence of leucocytes will make the diagnosis obvious, even if typical symptoms are not present. It is also important to consider the possibility of an underlying cause since urinary tract infections, particularly if recurrent, may be caused or exacerbated by underlying pathology.

Having excluded contamination or a lower urinary tract infection, the next step is to consider those conditions associated with chronic renal failure. If chronic renal failure is present there may be other evidence of renal damage in the urine, for instance casts and red and white blood cells, in addition to the biochemical markers of impaired renal function described above.

Although it occurs uncommonly in older people, the nephrotic syndrome is also a cause of proteinuria. It may occur more frequently than is generally appreciated. Although it may be due to minimal change lesions which will respond to treatment with prednisolone, it is more usually a concomitant of systemic diseases such as diabetes mellitus, collagenoses, malignancy, and more rarely renal vein thrombosis. A degree of nephrotic syndrome may accompany chronic congestive cardiac failure. This condition, i.e. nephrotic syndrome should be excluded in a patient presenting with heavy proteinuria, peripheral oedema, and hypoproteinaemia. The serum cholesterol may also be elevated. Hospital referral is indicated if it is suspected.

Asymptomatic bacteriuria

This is not an infrequent finding in elderly people and can pose problems in deciding whether or not treatment is appropriate. It is commonly associated with chronic pyleonephritis, and most authorities would probably agree that treatment is unnecessary unless symptoms develop or renal function is deteriorating. This is also true of the catheterized patient, although few doctors would dispute the value of attempting to treat it when it is first discovered. Repeated courses of antibiotics may, however, be more harmful than beneficial.

SUBDURAL HAEMATOMA

This is a condition which is commonly diagnosed at postmortem, since although the symptoms may be apparent shortly following an obvious injury, it is extremely common for the trauma responsible to be minor or forgotten and in the past. Classically it presents as fluctuating signs and symptoms, especially a fluctuating level of consciousness. Other presentations can include a fluctuating hemiplegia or other neurological signs, as well as more non-specific symptoms such as headache. As in the case of tuberculosis, subacute bacterial endocarditis and myxoedema, it is a condition for which a high index of suspicion must always be maintained when dealing with elderly patients and since treatment may result in considerable improvement, further investigation is always necessary. This is best arranged in the context of a short hospital admission which is often necessary in any case on account of the presenting disabilities. Where a patient is confined to a cottage hospital with radiological expertise a skull X-ray may reveal shift of mid-line structures and make the diagnosis more likely. If this is found, referral to the local neurosurgical centre is necessary for further confirmation and consideration of evacuation of the underlying haematoma if present. In any case in which there is doubt, hospital referral is necessary.

TEMPORAL ARTERITIS

Temporal arteritis is a condition which rarely occurs in younger people and has a peak incidence after the age of 55 to 60. Together with polymyalgia rheumatica it is considered by many authorities to be part of a spectrum of disease with considerable potential morbidity in the elderly. The arteritis may affect arteries other than the temporal artery, and even extracranial vessels. It classically presents with a throbbing temporal headache associated with scalp tenderness noticed when brushing or combing the hair. It may also present with complications such as blindness and localized neurological signs. If the temporal arteries are affected they will be found to be thickened and tender and to exhibit reduced pulsation. The occipital arteries can also be felt in this way in some people in whom they are affected. The more local symptoms and signs are usually accompanied by constitutional disability with a fever and malaise.

Diagnosis

The diagnosis is supported by finding a high ESR, especially if it is elevated above 100, but can only be definitively confirmed with a temporal artery biopsy. Unfortunately this may be unhelpful since occasionally there are skip lesions in the distribution of the arteritis and an apparently normal segment of artery may be excised. In addition it does not always affect the temporal arteries as mentioned previously.

Treatment

Treatment should never be delayed simply on the grounds of first obtaining a temporal artery biopsy. The risk of blindness or other occlusive arteritic event is sufficiently severe to warrant the immediate prescription of steroids, e.g. 40 to 60 mg of prednisolone daily. This is eventually reduced to the dose required to control the symptoms and maintain the ESR at an acceptable level. Five to ten milligrams a day usually suffice and should be continued for two years and then cautiously withdrawn with close monitoring of the patients symptoms and the ESR level. It must also be remembered that a recurrence may take the form not of temporal arteritis, but also of polymyalgia rheumatica. Any patient in whom temporal arteritis is considered to be present should be referred to hospital as an emergency.

THYROID DISORDERS

Hypothyroidism

Although all doctors know that myxoedema is often non-specific in its presentation in older patients and is therefore easily missed, the diagnosis is still not made in many cases and may elude even the keenest geriatrician or general physician. In the elderly it most commonly follows previous thyroid ablation or occurs as an idiopathic condition. The iatrogenic type may either be after surgery, when it is said that nearly 50 per cent of patients become myxoedematous within a year of partial thyroidectomy, or after radioactive iodine therapy when 80 per cent of patients are said to become myxoedematous within 15 years. The incidence is therefore very high following either procedure on the thyroid gland and should really be watched for rather than merely being picked up somewhat opportunistically.

Other causes of myxoedema include overdosage with antihyperthyroid drugs, as well as from other non-related compounds, e.g. lithium carbonate and the sulphonylureas. Hypopituitarism is rare in the elderly, and also auto-immune thyroiditis too. Nevertheless these conditions should be considered if it is not possible to explain the thyroid malfunction on other grounds. Auto-immune thyroiditis should particularly be considered if there is already a pre-existing auto-immune disorder such as pernicious anaemia, Addison's disease (of the idiopathic type), or vitiligo, whilst hypopituitarism is usually associated with evidence of loss of other trophic hormones. In both the latter, hospital referral is necessary for confirmation of the diagnosis.

Clinical features

These are the same in any age and do not merit detailed consideration here. There are, however, one or two points that are worth emphasizing. In the first place some of the classic features of myxoedema are a normal finding in many of the elderly, e.g. loss of the outer third of the eyebrows, and constipation, but they should nevertheless alert one to look for other signs. Particularly useful are the bradycardia in a patient who is not being treated concurrently with beta-blockers or some other drugs which could produce this, and the slowly relaxing reflexes. It must be stressed that it is the relaxation phase that is important and although it is usual to seek this sign with the ankle jerk, the biceps are often better in older people.

Investigations

Diagnosis can only be confirmed biochemically and the most useful investigation is the serum concentration of thyroxine (T4). The T3 level is unhelpful since a failing thyroid gland will often secrete more T3 than normal. If the T4 is reported as being within the borderline range the thyroid-stimulating hormone level (TSH) should be estimated and if elevated confirms the diagnosis. Occasionally, however, one is still uncertain after these tests and at this point it is probably best to refer the patient to hospital for a TRH test (thyrotrophin releasing hormone test), although this could be undertaken from general practice.

Thyroid hormone levels may be altered by other factors, such as oestrogen therapy, phenothiazine administration if this is prolonged, and in hypo-proteinaemic states since 99 per cent of the hormones are protein bound. If the TSH level is elevated, but the T4 level is within the normal range, it is not always necessary to conclude that the patient has myxoedema, since the TSH may be elevated in an attempt to 'drive' a failing thyroid gland. Under these circumstances the patient should be carefully followed up since there is a higher risk of hypothyroidism, and this is particularly so if there has been previous treatment for thyrotoxicosis.

Treatment

When treating the elderly for myxoedema it is *essential* to start with the lowest possible dose of thyroxine, and never more than 0.05 mg a day. They are very sensitive to exogenous thyroxine and there is always a risk of precipitating a myocardial infarction. Thyroxine takes three to four days to begin work with maximum response after a further week or so. Assuming that the initial dose is tolerated, it can be doubled at two-week intervals until a maximum of 0.2 mg a day is being taken. Very occasionally 0.3 mg will be necessary, but the correct dose is that which returns the T4 and TSH to normal values. It can then be monitored on clinical symptoms and signs, e.g. weight loss, tachycardia, heat intolerance, etc., and the T3 (triiodothyronine) level estimated if there is any evidence of early thyrotoxicosis. Since this is often a test which takes a week or two before the answer is available, it is probably best to ease back a little on the thyroxine dosage if there is objective clinical evidence of thyrotoxicosis.

Thyrotoxicosis

As is the case with myxoedema, thyrotoxicosis does not always present in the elderly with classical symptoms and signs. Indeed it is possible for the initial presentation to be one of apathy. Both the serum triiodothyronine (T3) and thyroxine (T4) are raised in most patients who are thyrotoxic, although some patients may have T3 thyrotoxicosis only and an even smaller number an elevation of thyroxine alone. An estimation of the T3 level by a radioimmunoassay technique is probably the best means of diagnosing the majority of thyrotoxic patients. It is also helpful in indicating which patients are relapsing into thyrotoxicosis after being treated.

The thyrotrophin-releasing hormone (TRH) test is occasionally necessary when investigating thyroid disease. Although this is usually performed in a hospital outpatient department, there is no reason why it could not be done in the general practitioner's surgery in the few cases where it is necessary. After blood has been taken to allow the basal TSH level to be measured, 200 microgrammes of TRH are injected intravenously and blood samples taken for subsequent estimations of TSH level 20 and 60 minutes after the injection. There is normally a peak response at about 20 minutes, but this is supressed in thyrotoxicosis since the raised level of thyroid hormones in the blood inhibit the release of TSH. This response, however, may also be affected by certain drugs, including L-dopa, corticosteroids, and also thyroxine if the dose is above 0.2 mg daily. Abnormal pituitary function will also prevent a response to the injection.

It is probably best to treat elderly people with thyrotoxicosis by medical means in the first instance, or with radioactive iodine and subsequent thyroid hormone replacement. In addition, many of the features of thyrotoxicosis will respond to treatment with beta-blockers, although they will have little affect on diarrhoea, weight loss, or eye signs. This can obviously be discontinued when the thyrotoxicosis has been brought under control.

TUBERCULOSIS

The dramatic drop in the incidence of tuberculosis in younger people has not been mirrored to the same extent in the elderly, mainly because so many of them have quiescent tuberculosis acquired in their youth. Reactivation of this primary infection is the commonest problem.

Presentation

This is often non-specific with ill-defined illness and general deterioration in health. It is easy to assume that it is secondary to an incurable wasting illness such as a neoplasm, which then makes further investigation of the patient less likely. It should therefore be considered a possibility in any patient with unexplained malaise, anorexia, weight loss and fever, as well as the more classical presentations such as persistent or recurrent chest infections and ascites.

A chest X-ray may help confirm the diagnosis, but all too often all one finds is the pre-existing changes indicating infection many years ago. Unless there is existing cavitation or miliary mottling, the chest X-ray may not be helpful. If a patient in whom tuberculosis is suspected is producing sputum, a sample should be sent for microscopy and culture and the possibility of tuberculosis specifically mentioned on the request card. It can also be helpful to re-X-ray a chest of doubtful significance six to eight weeks later in order to see if there has been any change if there are no previous X-rays with which to compare the present film.

Where the index of suspicion is high the patient should be referred to hospital for further investigation, and this should always be the case if there is a pleural effusion or ascites since these can be tapped and an appropriate specimen sent for microscopy and culture.

Tuberculin test

This is of doubtful value in the elderly since its interpretation is very difficult. Often a positive reaction only reflects previous infection rather than indicating present activity. The latter may be suspected if the reaction is extremely positive, however, but in so many cases it is not so. If the reaction is negative, active infection is unlikely unless the patient is the subject of an overwhelming infection which will be apparent on clinical grounds. A negative reaction in the presence of active disease also occurs in those who are immunosupressed, e.g. by drugs or a lymphoma. Occasionally, however, the reaction remains negative even in the presence of active infection. It is therefore preferable to diagnose active tuberculosis more objectively.

Treatment

This is similar to that in younger patients with one of the combination regimens. An effective combination consists of ethambutol for three months concurrently with isoniazid and rifampicin which are continued for six months or so after the ethambutol has been stopped. The three major worries in treating the elderly with tuberculosis are drug compliance with is often low, retrobulbar neuritis as a side-effect of ethambutol, and a need to avoid giving streptomycin if possible because of its high toxicity. These drugs are best prescribed initially under supervision in hospital.

VERTIGO/GIDDINESS/DIZZINESS

These three symptoms are listed together since elderly people often have great difficulty in differentiating between them. They are also occasionally confused with the feeling of faintness, collapsing, and other synonyms. Before it is possible to elucidate any underlying cause, the doctor needs to know exactly what the patient is complaining of. Although it is by no means a counsel of perfection, it is easiest from a practical point of view to divide this problem into two different subgroups. In the first of these the patient experiences true vertigo with a rotational sensation, usually of the room or furniture going round him. In the other group this does not happen and the overwhelming sensation is one of instability, faintness, etc., but without any rotational component.

True vertigo

This can be produced simply by an accumulation of wax in the external auditory meatus, which is responsible more frequently than most people appreciate. Middle-ear disease is also occasionally the cause in an older person, but disease of the auditory nerve, inner ear, cerebellum, and brain stem are probably commoner underlying factors. Brain stem territory cerebrovascular disease is probably the commonest cause, with labyrinthitis and Menière's disease following next. In the last-named there is paroxsymal labyrinthine disorder manifested as vertigo, deafness and vomiting accompanied by tinnitus. Many other pathologies in this area, however, may be responsible and this includes drug side-effects, e.g. over-dosage with Aspirin. Since occasionally more sinister but remediable conditions such as an acoustic neuroma can present in this way, it is important to obtain a further opinion if a diagnosis cannot be made easily or the symptoms do not respond to the appropriate treatment.

Giddiness/Dizziness, etc.

As described above, this implies the absence of any rotational sensation, which is usually the case, but unfortunately not always so. Vasovagal syncopal attacks occur in older people and occasionally for no reason, but before assuming this it is important to exclude hypotension whether postural or not, and anaemia. These pathologies always need further investigation. As in the case of true vertigo, disease of the brain stem, cerebellum, auditory nerve, and inner ear may also be involved.

In many cases no underlying cause for the problem is ever elucidated, and in some it improves spontaneously. Although a few of these cases may have had a self-limiting condition such as a short attack of labyrinthitis, one is forced to accept the fact that little is presently understood about one of the more common disabling symptoms of the elderly. If the symptoms persist in a patient in whom there is no obvious underlying cause, he or she must be counselled on the need to take care when making a turn or other rotational movement, and when rising from the sitting or lying position. Many drugs are claimed to be of benefit and different regimes have different advocates. Experience shows, however, that different preparations seem to suit different patients for no objective reason, and although it is worth trying drugs such as antihistamines, mild phenothiazines, and betahistine, they should be discontinued if there is no objective evidence of improvement. This is particularly important because their side-effects may include phenomenona which may aggravate a patient's original symptom, e.g. adding postural hypotension to their original presenting complaint. Referral to a geriatric or ENT clinic is necessary if an underlying condition is discovered which warrants this, or if troublesome symptoms persist.

Tinnitis is a common symptom which is often associated with vertigo, and can be extremely distressing. In excess of one in ten elderly people suffer with this problem at some stage. Referral for a further opinion is usually necessary, but often the only treatment possible is reassurance. This will help some sufferers, however, who associate it with an impending disaster, such as a stroke or inevitable deafness, but unfortunately many others have to learn to tolerate it. Serious consideration should always be given to the underlying cause, since it may be the first sign of potentially treatable pathology, e.g. Menière's disease and otosclerosis.

VISUAL IMPAIRMENT

There are so many potential causes of visual impairment in older people that it is not intended to try and cover them all, but rather to mention briefly those points which should be considered especially in more elderly patients. There are two approaches to the consideration of loss of sight, either using a structure by structure appraisal starting at the front of the eyeball and working backwards, or the more practical clinical approach which will be used here. This divides the visual impairment into two major types, acute and chronic.

Acute loss of vision

Acute loss of vision is obviously an ophthalmological emergency. Severe pain in the eyes associated with vomiting in many instances and blurred vision from corneal oedema probably heralds an acute attack of angle closure glaucoma. This should be further suspected if an oval dilated pupil fails to respond to light. In many patients there will have been previous subacute but self limiting attacks.

Immediate referral to an eye hospital casualty department is necessary for intensive pilocarpine and acetazolamide therapy or other medical treatment, and in the majority of cases probably drainage surgery.

Useful advice for old people and their relatives on sight

Warning signs that need medical attention the same day

1. Persistent pain.
2. Sensitivity to light.
3. Seeing halos and rainbows around lights.
4. Flashing lights.
5. Loss of vision.
6. Double vision.
7. Redness and irritation.

There are especially two retinal conditions which are associated with the sudden loss of vision. One of these is the detached retina and the other occlusive vascular disease affecting either the arterial or the venous system. Both require urgent ophthalmological assessment and should be referred to an Eye Department without delay. The history, e.g. features of temporal arteritis or glaucoma, and examination of the eye, e.g. the retinal palor and 'cherry red spot' of central or branch retinal arterial occlusion will often indicate what has occurred. However, the finer points of diagnosis and consideration of any underlying predisposing pathological entities is best left to the hospital.

Sometimes a patient claims to have lost vision in one or other eye when the lesion is really within the brain. The most frequent reason for this is probably the sudden onset of a homonymous hemi-anopia, which is interpreted by the patient as being caused by loss of sight in one or other eye. This may occur as a consequence of a cerebrovascular accident when full examination will often reveal other localizing neurological signs, even if only of a mild nature. If any doubt exists however, a second opinion is necessary.

Chronic loss of vision

Slow onset of visual impairment is met with more frequently in older people than the acute and more urgent problems described above.

Cataract

Cataract formation is common, and although in many people no underlying factors can be discovered, it is important to consider these, e.g. diabetes mellitus and long-term steroid therapy. If the cataract is unilateral and the other eye has normal or adequate vision, it is not necessary to consider cataract extraction unless there are other relevant factors, such as the onset of secondary glaucoma and other less common conditions in the elderly. Cataract removal should be considered when vision is impaired to the extent that the activities of daily living are significantly affected, although the introduction of many modern techniques has resulted in a trend towards earlier surgical treatment.

Retinopathy

Retinopathy, especially that of diabetes, is often discovered as an incidental finding when examining the fundus. In many patients, however, it contributes to visual impairment, as does the retinopathy of hypertension, although this is probably not so prevalent amongst the elderly. Both should indicate the need for careful control of the underlying condition, and in the case of diabetic retinopathy, xenon arc or laser coagulation are occasionally used. Macular degeneration typically appearing as coarse dark mottling in the macular area has no specific treatment, but it is worth recommending the use of a magnifying glass for reading, and/or strong reading glasses. Often, however, the patient has discovered this for themselves.

Chronic glaucoma

Chronic glaucoma can also lead to loss of vision and can either be the result of open angle glaucoma, i.e. raised intraocular pressure unassociated with obstruction to the filtration angle of the iris, or a chronic form of the closed angle variety. Until the visual loss is noted by the patient, these conditions may remain asymptomatic and the prolonged rise in pressure will lead to a visual field defect and a pathological degree of cupping of the optic disc. This of course needs hospital referral when suspected for supervision of medical treatment and consideration of drainage surgery if necessary.

It can be seen that careful examination of the eye is as important in the more chronic type of visual deterioration as it is in the case of acute loss of vision. It is also necessary to remember that in an old person more than one pathology may be responsible for the deficit. Since sight, together with preservation of mobility and intellectual capacity, is one of the major bastions of independence, it is extremely important to take seriously any complaint by a patient of loss of vision. In addition, since this section has attempted to cover only a few common situations arising in older people, the reader is referred to standard ophthalmological texts and to the need for specialist advice should the situation warrant it.

Blindness and mental health

There is evidence that blindness can affect mental health in old age. The following symptoms may develop as a result of blindness:

Anxiety.

Depression.

Confusion, which usually results from isolation, but sensory deprivation can cause confusion even if the older person is not isolated.

These are not inevitable consequences of blindness, but develop if the old person and his relatives are not helped to adjust to the loss of vision.

Help for blind and partially sighted people

Because of the low expectations of elderly people and their relatives many older patients with visual impairment do not receive sufficient help. It is often assumed that nothing can be done to treat the cause of the visual problem or to investigate its effects. In addition for many elderly people their visual problem is not the most significant. One survey found that only 56 per cent of visually impaired old people counted poor sight among their greatest troubles. It has been estimated that the Blind Register only contains the names of two thirds of blind elderly people, although 90 per cent of them are in contact with their general practitioner.

Registration is important because it brings some practical benefits, but the main benefit is that it brings the old person into contact with the social worker for the blind, who is able to advise the older person and his relatives. The social worker for the blind is based either in the eye hospital or in the social services department and works closely with two new types of professional worker:

(a) The mobility officer who is trained to help a blind person regain the ability to move about outside his home in confidence and safety.

(b) The rehabilitation officer who helps the blind person regain the ability to look after himself and his home.

Unfortunately there are very few of these workers, so much of the support is left to the relatives of the blind person. There are a number of important points to emphasize to relatives:

Help the old person make the most of the vision he has by keeping his spectacles clear and by ensuring regular checks at the opticians if he is not attending a hospital clinic. If ordinary spectacles are a problem the hospital clinic will be able to advise on low-vision aids such as magnifying glasses.

Improve domestic lighting by putting in more powerful bulbs and moving lights closer to where the old person sits and reads.

Try to encourage mental stimulation by arranging for volunteers to bring large print books or cassettes from the library. The telephone and radio also offer very useful stimulation. The social worker for the blind will be able to advise about the telephones for the blind and wireless for the blind charities.

Try to prevent isolation if the old person lives alone by encouraging him to go out. The social worker or mobility officer should be consulted if isolation appears to be developing. Adjustment to blindness may be helped by attending a club run specially for blind people.

In addition relatives also need advice on two other important aspects of blindness – communication and mobility:

Advice for relatives on communication

Always let a blind person know when you are approaching.

Introduce yourself every time.

Hold his hand if he finds it helps him locate the position of your face.

Remember that blind people lose a great deal of what is going on by missing non-verbal cues, notably when they wish to enter a conversation. More formal verbal cues such as a question which includes the blind person, name, etc. are therefore necessary. When a number of people are present the old person can be told to raise his hand if he finds it difficult to break in.

Always announce that you are leaving clearly and leave quickly after saying good-bye.

Useful advice for old people and their relatives

Mobility

1. When guiding a blind person let him take your arm; do not grab him and try to steer him.
2. Let the blind person walk a little way behind you, about half a pace or so; do not push him in front. Tell him about obstacles before you reach them.
3. Always approach steps and kerbs at right angles.
4. To help him enter a car, place one hand on the roof above the open door and the other on the top of the door. When helping him to sit down do not try to reverse him into the chair; put his hand on the back of the chair and let him find his own way.

If the old person or his relatives are having difficulty, the mobility officer or social worker for the blind should be able to help.

WEIGHT LOSS

Many elderly people seem to lose weight without passing comment on this fact. Consistent weight loss, however, is a symptom of significance and should always be treated seriously. Unfortunately, it is a common facet of so many conditions that the aetiology is often difficult to unravel. As is usually the case, it is best to start with a history and examination since these will often indicate the most likely areas to pursue in more detail, although this is not always so and it is then necessary to tackle the problems step by step. The outline below covers the majority of the important causes of weight loss. Malnutrition is a common factor causing or contributing to weight loss in the elderly and is discussed on page 62: Malabsorption, occurring less frequently also requires consideration (p. 62). The other major causes of weight loss are described below.

Malignant disease of GI tract

A past history of pernicious anaemia, atrophic gastritis, or gastric ulceration indicates that the patient has a higher chance of developing a gastric carcinoma. This is a relatively common tumour in older people and weight loss is often the only symptom. Quite advanced neoplasms can present with little more than weight loss and a mild degree of anaemia. Unfortunately, the majority of patients with this condition are suffering with advanced disease by the time they present, even though the symptoms and signs are so minimal. Major surgery is rarely undertaken, but palliative operative measures can significantly improve the quality of life in an elder with an advanced growth if they are suffering from uncomfortable symptoms. In the majority of cases the diagnosis will be confirmed by the barium meal, although it is often best to have histological confirmation of this. In the latter case, or when a barium meal is unhelpful, gastroscopy is important and the patient should be referred to hospital for this purpose.

If the weight loss is accompanied by dysphagia, a malignancy in the oesophagus must be considered, although a carcinoma in the fundus of the stomach, or indeed a benign stricture at the bottom of the oesophagus are also important causes. The investigations are the same as for a suspected carcinoma of the stomach.

Weight loss associated with rectal bleeding, or a disturbance of bowel function should be treated in the same way in an older person as in a younger patient, namely with a sigmoidoscopy and barium enema. It is important not to assume that these symptoms indicate a definite neoplasm and that age is a contra-indication for surgery. The elderly are of course prone to the same non-malignant conditions which cause this symptomatology in young people and for which treatment can be very rewarding.

Peptic ulceration

A chronic peptic ulcer often leads to weight loss, but in some people the high milk intake resorted to for symptomatic relief can actually result in weight gain. This, however, is unusual and certainly will not be relevant in a person who is complaining of weight loss. The same measures are adopted in older people as in their younger counterparts when dealing with peptic ulcers. These include carbenoxolone sodium, although care must be taken that the resulting salt and water retention and hypokalaemia do not aggravate pre-existing cardiac failure, or a tendency in this direction. Anticholinergic drugs are rarely used in the elderly because they are known to precipitate urinary retention, to aggravate constipation and to cause a rise in intraocular pressure.

One of the most effective drugs in many patients is Cimetidine, but difficulties can ensue when the time has come to discontinue it, and it is probably best to tail it off when the course has finished rather than to abruptly stop the patient taking it.

It is also very important to remember that a gastric ulcer which does not heal after an adequate trial of therapy should be biopsied in case it is malignant.

Carcinoma of the pancreas

This neoplasm is common in the elderly and is often found to be the cause of a painless obstructive jaundice. It may, however, present as weight loss with little else to indicate its presence. It is then very difficult to diagnose and not infrequently remains unsuspected until further symptoms develop. A carcinoma of the head of the pancreas is often associated with epigastric pain which characteristically often radiates into the back and may be relieved by leaning forward. This is a very difficult neoplasm to remove surgically, but if obstruction to the biliary tree results, a patient's quality of life can often be considerably improved with the help of palliative surgery, such as a by-pass procedure. This may change a miserable outlook to one in which the patient can live a meaningful existence for several months before he dies. If this condition is suspected it is probably best to refer the patient to a surgical or gastro-enterological outpatient department for further investigation.

Endocrine conditions

Although diabetes mellitus and thyrotoxicosis can both cause weight loss in older people, thyrotoxicosis is the less common of the two and often presents in an atypical manner. Diabetes should of course be suspected if there is a history of increasing thirst and polyuria, often most strikingly manifested as nocturia. as well as weight loss. Often, however, the symptoms are not volunteered, or are misrepresented in such a way that they are considered to be indicative of another pathology, for instance a urinary tract infection. The symptoms are very similar to those in younger people, although more frequently than in the latter the patient presents in coma or pre-coma since so many elderly people live on their own with nobody to report their illness, or urge them to seek further attention. Thyrotoxicosis can present as an apathetic patient with atrial fibrillation, a goitre, and weight loss, rather than the more typical presentation with hyperactivity seen in younger people. The diagnosis of both these conditions and their management is along the same lines as in younger people and treatment is further discussed elsewhere (diabetes, p. 38; thyrotoxicosis, p. 78).

Psychiatric disease

Depression can present with weight loss and is easy to miss. When diagnosed it must be remembered that many of the drugs normally prescribed are likely to precipitate side-effects in older people. If treatment is difficult or unsatisfactory, the patient should be referred for a psychogeriatric opinion. Where appropriate, it is often more satisfactory for the patient to undergo a course of ECT than a prolonged course of antidepressants.

The other common psychiatric cause of weight loss is dementia. Senile dementia is considered at length elsewhere (p. 28), but unless there is a treatable cause for the intellectual deterioration, there is little that can or should be done about the weight loss of terminal dementia.

Other conditions

A malignancy anywhere may cause weight loss. Other common tumours in addition to those already mentioned include bronchus, breast, lymphomas, and leukaemias. If a neoplasm is suspected it is best to attempt to define only those that may be treatable or open to the possibility of amelioration. An extensive and exhaustive hunt for a primary malignancy should not be taken in an older patient unless there is a good cause.

Cryptic infection is not an uncommon cause of illness discovered at post mortem. In particular, the elderly are subject to subacute bacterial endocarditis and tuberculosis, both of which may present in a variety of ways and may not be discovered until after the patient has died. Although the investigations are the same as in a patient of a younger age, a very high index of suspicion is needed in the elderly since these conditions and other cryptic infections often respond well to treatment.

Drugs as a cause of weight loss resulting from malabsorption have already been mentioned. Many other drugs, however, can also produce weight loss, for instance by causing anorexia. One of the commonest is Digoxin, which should always be prescribed with caution, and the need for continued therapy reviewed from time to time.

A systematic approach to the problem of weight loss will often result in the elucidation of the underlying disease. In many instances, hospital referral is unnecessary for either investigation or management.

Weight loss check-list

Could the cause of the weight loss be:
1. Deficient intake (see p. 62)?
2. Dental problems?
3. Dysphagia?
4. Malabsorption?
5. Peptic ulceration?
6. Neoplasm of stomach; large bowel; pancreas; elsewhere?
7. Diabetes?
8. Thyrotoxicosis?
9. Tuberculosis or other chronic infection?
10. Depression?

4 Prescribing for the elderly

The principles of prescribing for the elderly are similar to those in younger patients, that is, is the drug required at all and if so is this the right preparation in the correct dose; are the side-effects going to be worse than the therapeutic benefits; is this the best type of preparation (e.g. liquid versus capsule) and can the old person read the label and instructions easily; and probably most importantly, when am I going to review the need to continue prescribing this drug? Although these principles are similar in all ages there are many details which are different and extremely important to bear in mind at all times. Some of the more important are discussed below.

Older people are more susceptible to adverse reactions and one has to strike the balance between morbidity from side-effects and a therapeutic gain. This is particularly so in some drugs where the margin between therapeutic benefit and the problems of toxicity is very narrow, e.g. in the treatment of cardiological and neurological conditions such as cardiac failure and parkinsonism.

It is best if, where practical, one doctor is primarily responsible for all the prescribing for an individual elderly patient. In this way some of the hazards of polypharmacy may be avoided. In one study recently (Williamson 1978) it was discovered that 80 per cent of those admitted to geriatric wards were receiving drug treatment of one sort or another and 25 per cent of patients over 75 years old were receiving three or more drugs on a regular basis. Having one doctor principally involved in prescribing for each patient may also avoid the risk of repeat prescriptions being signed without adequate review of the need to do so.

COMPLIANCE

The study of compliance rightly, albeit belatedly, has been one of the growth areas of modern medicine. Two excellent reviews of compliance have recently been published – *Compliance in health care,* and *Compliance with therapeutic regimes,* edited by Sackett and Haynes (1976), which was published three years earlier. In addition a number of reviews of compliance among older patients have been published.

In spite of the methodological problems in this area of research four factors are generally agreed to be associated with good compliance and a low rate of problems:

The simplicity of the regime.
The absence of side-effects or the need to change one's life-style.
Clear and appropriate information.
The quality of the doctor–patient relationship.

Simple regimes

A simple regime contains as few drugs as possible in the simplest regime possible for the shortest time possible.

Adverse effects of treatment

If treatment has adverse effects on the patient, either drug side-effects or a major change in life-style, the probability that compliance will be poor is increased. Some treatments inevitably involve side-effects or change in life-style, but every effort should be made to minimize them. The need for careful follow-up is obvious and widely appreciated, but many problems still occur because insufficient attention is paid to the review of long-term medication. This is not to argue that repeat prescriptions should never be issued without seeing the patient but it is necessary to work out a system which allows for the review of elderly people on long-term medication at a frequency which is appropriate to each case.

Clear and appropriate information

The instructions given to the patient should obviously be clear. They should obviously be set in words and terms familiar to the old person and if written instructions are given they should be printed in type big enough for the old person to be able to read it – typewriter capitals are a good size and lines should be double-spaced. It is, however, also important that the information is appropriate to the patient's beliefs about his disease and treatment.

The incorporation of the patient's beliefs about disease and treatment into his education has been called the 'health belief' approach and it has been shown to be effective in influencing patients and improving compliance. The beliefs that must be taken into account when educating a patient are his beliefs about:

(a) the seriousness of the disease 'Does it cause serious disability or only minor inconvenience?';

(b) his personal susceptibility to the unpleasant consequences of the disease: 'Is it one in a million or one in ten that I could be seriously affected?';

(c) the benefits of therapy: 'Will the treatment work, or am I too old for treatment?'.

Advice has therefore to be based not only on pharmacological evidence but on the patient's own beliefs and attitudes, and, as we have already emphasized, these are particularly important when treating older people because many older people assume that they are suffering from the effects of aging which they know to be inevitable and untreatable when they are in effect suffering from the effects of a treatable disease.

The doctor–patient relationship

Because of the scientific rigour of modern professors and editors and those who dispense research funds most research workers focus on those aspects of medicine which can be measured, counted, and chi-squared. Valuable though this approach has been, it has meant that these aspects of medicine which did not lend themselves to measurement, counting, or statistics have been relatively ignored and one of these is the quality of the doctor–patient relationship, but there is good evidence that the quality of the relationship is an important determinant of good compliance and of course general practitioners have, in general, a good relationship with their elderly patients. Because of this, Dr James Knox argued in a very useful review of *Prescribing for the elderly in general practice* that 'the magnitude of the problem had been overestimated because many of the studies had been hospital based. The doctor who is interested in his patient's beliefs and sensitive to his fears will achieve better compliance than the doctor who is, or appears to be, less interested.'

PHARMACOKINETICS AND PHARMACODYNAMICS

Pharmacokinetics and pharmacodynamics differ in older patients and this will have a bearing on the dosage of many drugs. Factors such as the different distribution of drugs within different body compartments, impaired metabolism, and renal clearance and altered sensitivity to some drugs, e.g. an increase in sensitivity to nitrazepam and a decrease for beta-blockers further complicate the issue. In general where there is any doubt it is better to err on the side of giving too low a dose.

POLYPHARMACY

The most important point to consider in prescribing for an older patient is when to review the benefit or otherwise that the patient is experiencing. Polypharmacy often originates simply because of a failure of the prescriber to consider discontinuing a course of treatment.

The remainder of this chapter will discuss some of the pit-falls and problems associated with some of the drugs prescribed for older people. It does not contain an exhaustive list of side-effects, and nor is it meant to, but is designed to bring to the attention of the reader problems which are commonly encountered and which should be considered before prescribing the preparations in question.

HYPNOTICS

Before prescribing a hypnotic it is important to be clear in one's mind why it is required, and to try alternative means of producing sleep before prescribing a drug. Sometimes the problem identified by the old person is not a problem which requires treatment. Some old people become anxious that they are not sleeping as well as they were without appreciating that their decreased levels of physical and mental activity and their daytime naps reduce the need for sleep at

> **Useful advice for old people and their relatives**
>
> *Preventing sleeping problems*
>
> The most important means of preventing or treating sleeping problems is to establish a pattern of behaviour which will be followed every evening, for example:
>
> 9.30 p.m. A warm drink, such as Horlicks, Ovaltine, or Cocoa, not tea or coffee, or a night-cap if there are no contra-indications. This should be taken sitting in the same chair, perhaps with music playing but no television after 9 p.m.
>
> 9.45 p.m. Bath.
>
> 10.15 p.m. Read some soothing book or magazine, not a thriller.
>
> 10.30 p.m. Go to a bed which should be warm and well made.
>
> 10.45 p.m. Lights out.

night. Sometimes the anxiety about sleeplessness becomes the main factor perpetuating the the sleeplessness (Fig. 4.1).

In trying to sleep better, the old person who is anxious about his sleeping may try a number of different approaches and this in turn increases the problem because an established pre-sleep ritual is a very important means of promoting sleep, and the old person should be encouraged to try to re-establish a set sequence of events before he goes to bed before a hypnotic drug is prescribed.

Sleeplessness may be the result of remediable problems such as ischaemic limb pain, nocturia, orthopnea, depression, etc. The hypnotic may be necessary in addition to treatment for another condition, and if so one must remember to discontinue the hypnotic when the underlying condition has been treated. The benzodiazepines are probably the most widely prescribed hypnotic and the starting dose should be half that used in younger patients. Where possible it is

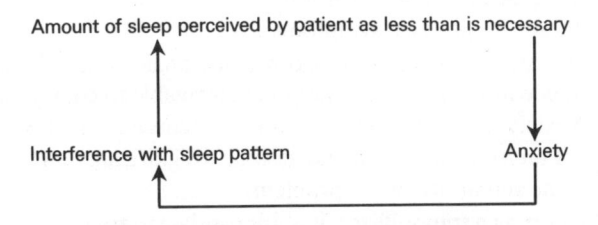

Fig. 4.1. The vicious cycle of insomnia.

probably best to use one of the shorter-acting drugs, e.g. temazepam. If a benzodiazepine is inappropriate, chlormethiazole is a useful alternative.

TRANQUILLIZERS

Tranquillizers may be used to lessen the level of agitation without making the patient drowsy. As with hypnotics it is important to discover why the patient is agitated in case the cause of the agitation also requires treatment. Phenothiazines of the chlorpromazine type should be avoided wherever possible and a small dose of a benzodiazepine, e.g. oxazepam or mild phenothiazine such as thioridazine tried instead. A small dose of haloperidol or chlormethiazole may also be useful, especially for maintenance treatment.

Whatever the dose of phenothiazine or haloperidol, side-effects such as parkinsonism, tardive dyskinesia, drowsiness, and postural hypotension must be watched for. In the case of phenothiazines especially, hypothermia and cholestatic jaundice may occur.

There are many potential contributory factors to anxiety, alleviation of which may obviate the need for drug treatment.

The principal cause of anxiety is uncertainty and there are many uncertainties in old age. Some of the more common are:

Will I have to go and live in a home?
Will I develop dementia?
Will I become a burden on my family?
Will I fall again?
Will I be incontinent again?
Will I be able to pay my fuel bills?
Will I be mugged?

These are only a few of the more common causes of anxiety. The old person may complain of anxiety but it may present in other ways, or be referred by relatives without mention of anxiety. Anxiety may cause:

Weight loss.
Alcohol abuse.
Neglect of self or environment.
Agitation or restlessness, or confusion.
Preoccupation with physical symptoms.

Patients who are demented may also become anxious and the management of anxiety is made more difficult if the person is unable to communicate why he is anxious. Anxiety is aggravated by isolation because a small worry can prey on the mind of an isolated person and assume a significance which is out of all proportion to the actual size of the problem.

Before prescribing a tranquillizer, it is appropriate to try to give simple advice to the elderly person and his relatives.

Useful advice for old people and their relatives

Helping to control anxiety

1. No matter how trivial the matter seems take time to discuss it.
2. When listening look calm and confident and do not be afraid to hold the person's hand to reassure him while talking to him.
3. Do not just say 'don't worry', take some positive step to reduce the cause of the anxiety, if the older person can identify a cause.
4. Suggest that the priest call, if the old person is religious. Prayer is often very helpful.
5. Try to reduce the old person's isolation.
6. Inform the general practitioner of the anxiety if it lasts for days, or if it intrudes into every thought or conversation, or if it is not allayed by solving the problem which the old person has identified as the cause of his anxiety.

DIURETICS

Loop diuretics, i.e. those acting on the loop of Henle, are usually unnecessary in elderly people as maintenance therapy for cardiac failure or hypertension. Milder diuretics are preferable, e.g. the thiazides. The loop diuretics most commonly used are frusemide and bumetanide. They can cause such a profound diuresis with alterations in plasma volume and plasma electrolyte levels that many patients experience severe side-effects, especially hypotension, as well as the social embarrassment of needing to make frequent visits to the toilet.

Potassium supplements are necessary in the majority of patients on diuretics, unless they are taking a potassium sparing compound such as spironolactone, amiloride, or triamterene. It is not adequate to just measure the serum potassium level since 200–300 mmol of potassium may be lost before there is any fall in a serum level. Plasma urea and electrolytes should probably be checked at least every six months in patients on long-term diuretic therapy. In many patients a soluble form of potassium is preferable to tablets.

It should be remembered that thiazides can aggravate or precipitate hyperuricaemia and diabetes, and that diuretics should rarely be prescribed for ankle oedema unless this is caused by heart failure.

DIGOXIN

Digoxin is rarely indicated in elderly patients in sinus rhythm. The major indication for prescribing it is the patient with atrial fibrillation and mitral valve disease. Very few patients need digoxin because of heart failure in other circumstances.

This drug is renally cleared from the body and therefore affected by the decreased renal clearance which is present in so many of our elders. Loading doses should never be more than 0.5 to 1 mg in divided doses over 24 hours and in many patients a maintenance dose as little as 0.0625 mg will be sufficient.

In theory it is best to check on the following before prescribing digoxin – serum potassium and urea levels, and an ECG to exclude conditions such as heart block, and ventricular dysrrhythmias including multiple ectopics.

Overdosage in the elderly is common and manifested by symptoms such as nausea, vomiting, anorexia, diarrhoea, confusion and disturbance of cardiac rhythm, as well as the more classical xanthopsia.

ANTIHYPERTENSIVES

Many older people are unnecessarily treated for hypertension, although the necessity for any treatment in those aged 70 years or more is considered by many to be controversial. In general, it is correct to treat an elderly person with a diastolic blood pressure in excess of 105–110 mm of mercury when this has been discovered on more than one occasion. A time may also come when we will recognize the need to treat elderly patients with systolic hypertension (which is currently under review). Treatment of hypertensive patients with a diastolic of less than 105–110 mm Hg is also necessary when there is evidence of target organ damage, such as retinopathy, and cardiological and renal impairment.

It is probably best to start with a diuretic, adding a beta-blocker if necessary. Some doctors prefer to use hydrallazine or methyldopa, but the latter is not usually prescribed as first-line treatment any more. Drugs that should specifically be avoided are guanethidine, bethanidine, debrisoquine, and reserpine. Occasionally a patient who has been controlled on one of these preparations for many years without adverse effects can continue with this treatment, but it should not be instituted in newly diagnosed cases.

DRUGS FOR PARKINSONISM

L-dopa combination preparations are gaining increasing acceptance as the front-line of treatment against Parkinson's disease. Before prescribing one of these drugs it is necessary to ensure that the parkinsonian symptoms are not the side-effects of other drugs, e.g. phenothiazines. Should this be the case then the preferred treatment would be to remove or decrease the dose of the phenothiazine, or prescribe an anticholinergic preparation, such as benzhexol or orphenadrine instead. An anticholinergic drug is probably also best in most patients in whom tremor is the major problem.

All the drugs used to treat parkinsonism have a very narrow margin of safety between the therapeutic effect and toxic levels. Common side-effects include confusion and hypotension, and the anticholinergic properties of some of them may precipitate glaucoma and urinary retention.

It is the author's opinion that when a combination preparation is necessary, a mixture of L-dopa and benserazide is less likely to produce gastro-intestinal tract side-effects and therefore is often better tolerated. This may reflect a different proportion of L-dopa to decarboxylase inhibitor in the existing preparations, rather than the pharmacological property of the substances themselves.

ANTIMICROBIALS

From the General Practice point of view the most important drug to avoid in the elderly, or use with caution, is probably tetracycline and its derivatives. Tetracyclines can raise the blood urea in patients with impaired renal function even to the extent of producing severe renal failure. These preparations are almost exclusively cleared from the body via the kidney and one should at least be certain that the patient has normal renal function before prescribing a tetracycline derivative.

The exception to this is doxycycline, which is mainly excreted through the bile and is therefore safe in the presence of renal failure. It has the added advantage of a single daily dosage compared to the t.d.s. or q.d.s. administration needed with the others.

DRUGS FOR DIABETES

Fortunately, few elderly patients require insulin, but when they do practical problems may make control of the blood-sugar level difficult. In particular, insulin is difficult to administer if the patient has arthritis in their hands or failing eyesight. The latter will also make it difficult for them to adequately assess the glycosuria they are producing. It may well be necessary to ask the district nurse or a relative to undertake this.

When a drug is being prescribed for maturity onset diabetes, most physicians use a sulphonylurea rather than a biguanide in the first instance. The short-acting sulphonylureas are preferable to the others such as chlopropamide since the long half-life of the latter coupled with its renal clearance has resulted in many instances of catastrophic hypoglycaemia. Sulphonylureas unfortunately make many patients feel hungry and consequently they may have difficulty in sticking to their diet. Dietary treatment in the elderly is in itself often unsatisfactory because food is one of the few pleasures left to an older person, but weight reduction should be tried.

If a biguanide is added to the drug regime, metformin should be used in preference to phenformin, and the potential hazards of lactic acidosis borne in mind. Biguanides are best used in combination with a sulphonylurea and are rarely satisfactory on their own.

ANTIDEPRESSANTS

Depression is the commonest mental problem in old age, and the causes for this are obvious. Depression is often aggravated by isolation and can become a problem when an old person feels it is a problem, but the old person may not complain of depression and it may present as:

Loss of appetite.
Constipation.
Neglect of self or surroundings.
Abuse of alcohol.
Agitation and restlessness, often referred as confusion.

Depression must always be considered as one of the alternative diagnoses to dementia as it can be missed. It is important to remember that the two diagnoses are not mutually exclusive. Both conditions may present:

Failure to take prescribed medication.
Immobility.

The suicide rate is higher in older age groups and consideration must always be given to the possibility that the older person is considering suicide. Often an older patient will say 'I just wish that I could just go to sleep and not wake up',

---

Useful advice for old people and their relatives

Helping a depressed person

1. Always pay serious attention to depression, even if the cause seems trivial. Seek professional help if you are worried or if the old person speaks of suicide.
2. Let the person talk about the cause of his depression; remember that it can be very comforting to hold a hand and put an arm round the depressed person's shoulders.
3. Try to encourage the depressed person to think of any aspects of his life which give him joy, such as a favourite grandchild; use photographs and tape recordings when appropriate.
4. Try to reduce the old person's isolation.
5. If he is religious, or used to attend Church regularly, ask the priest to call; prayer is an effective antidepressent.
6. Ask for help if these measures do not relieve the depression.

and a statement like this calls for question, 'do you feel like taking your own life?'. Usually the answer given by the old person is that suicide is wrong, but the answer to the question is occasionally in the affirmative, in which case prompt action must be taken. However, most people who are depressed can be helped by the support of friends, relatives, and professionals, supplemented sometimes by the judicious use of antidepressants.

Depressed elderly patients who do not respond to a course of tricyclic therapy should be referred to a psychogeriatrician for assessment. ECT in appropriate patients may avoid the need for a long course of treatment with tricyclic drugs and their attendant problems. The number of drugs for depression on the market is legion and it is important to start with the smallest possible dose, slowly increasing this as necessary. The most prominent side-effects of tricyclic compounds are usually those associated with the anticholinergic actions, and include a dry mouth, blurred vision, constipation, and more importantly urinary retention and disturbance of cardiac rhythm and rate. They are also potent producers of confusion and a well-known cause of postural hypotension.

Monoamine oxidase inhibitors are rarely used in the elderly, but the newer tetracyclic preparations may be worth trying.

5 The pattern of services

GERIATRIC HOSPITAL SERVICES

The pattern of geriatric hospital services is similar in many areas of the country, but there will of course be local differences in terms of the emphasis placed upon certain resources and the availability of some of the facilities, in part reflecting the economic situation and the relative importance or otherwise of the care of the elderly in the list of priorities of the local Health Authority.

Inpatient care

In many geriatric services the inpatient services are divided into three main types. The first type of geriatric bed is for the acute treatment and also for the assessment of ill elderly people. In theory, these beds should be in the main district general hospital with equal access to the same laboratory and supporting services as the acute beds for younger patients. Unfortunately in many areas even the acute geriatric beds are provided in a separate isolated hospital, in some instances without immediate access to laboratory investigations.

The second type of bed is that in an acute rehabilitation unit. These beds provide rehabilitation for an elderly patient after the acute medical side of their problem has been sorted out. In many geriatric services this type of rehabilitation bed is found in the same ward as the acute bed.

The majority of geriatric units separate those beds for slow-stream rehabilitation or continuing care patients from the other two streams of care. Although the majority of patients on a ward of this nature who have been labelled continuing care will spend the rest of their days in hospital, it must be noted that the adoption of this term implies that some will eventually become fit enough to return to the community. It is not uncommon for a patient to make sufficient a recovery to leave hospital after as long a period as a year to 18 months, and in some instances even longer.

Acutely ill elderly people, when accepted by the geriatric service, will usually be admitted direct into an acute geriatric bed. In many units patients can be admitted to either of the other types of care, but usually after they have been assessed either in the home, in the day hospital, or in an outpatient clinic.

Outpatient clinics

Many geriatric outpatient clinics take the form of an assessment clinic in which the elderly patient can be given an adequate amount of time to allow full assessment of both the medical and social problems which they are encountering. This type of clinic can therefore cope with complex medico-social situations, as well as the appropriate investigation of a purely medical problem. It is therefore appropriate to refer a patient with either type of problem to an assessment clinic.

The floating bed

This is an intermittent admission scheme enabling a patient to spend perhaps three days (two nights) every fortnight or a longer period at a greater interval in hospital so that their medical and social status can be assessed and their relatives or carers allowed the opportunity of having a break. This arrangement often allows a patient who might otherwise end up in a long-stay bed to remain in the community.

Holiday admission

This is an intermittent admission of longer duration, usually one or two weeks once or twice a year to enable relatives or carers to have a longer break, usually with the intention of permitting them the opportunity to have a proper holiday of their own. Holiday admissions are obviously much sought after at peak holiday times and in consequence it is essential to think ahead and make an application for a holiday bed early in the year.

The day hospital

There is a lot of confusion about the use of day hospitals. In general they are not there to provide a social outlet or in common parlance 'granny sitting service'. Attendance at day hospital implies a therapeutic need, either for rehabilitation or attention to a medical problem for instance. There are a few people, however, whose relatives need to be given a break during the week who attend day hospitals, but this is usually only if there is a medical problem that cannot be looked after by any of the other facilities providing day care.

Day hospitals are also used for the initial assessment of a patient where it is thought it would be more meaningful for them to be observed over a period of time rather than in the shorter period allowed in an outpatient clinic. A good day hospital has access to the same staff as an acute assessment ward since in many respects its functions are very similar, namely helping an elderly person to live in or return to the community.

Domiciliary visits

Domiciliary visits are usually undertaken for two major reasons. The first of these is in an attempt to maintain a patient in the community and prevent a hospital admission. It is extremely useful for the geriatrician to see the patient

102 *The pattern of services*

in his own environment in these circumstances. Even if admission does become necessary the knowledge gained will be invaluable in returning a patient to his own home if this is the eventual outcome.

The other major indication for a domiciliary visit is the patient who is obviously ill, but who does not wish to go into hospital. If adequately forewarned of this the geriatrician can arrive complete with syringes, specimen tubes, ECG, etc. In other words attempting to take the diagnostic service of the hospital to the patient.

It must be remembered that the major aim of the geriatric department is to enable the elderly people in its catchment area to be maintained at home as long as possible. This involves careful liaising with the community services and also with the general practitioner and his primary health care team. Unfortunately, many geriatric departments have an inadequate number of beds to cope with the potential workload, and at times the community finds itself very stretched in trying to look after, at home, people who may well be better off in hospital. As the numbers of the frail elderly, especially those aged 75 and over, increases in the next 20 years this is a situation that will become of greater concern to all.

Although many general practitioners will not find it necessary or desirable to undertake a visit to their local geriatric service upon taking up an appointment in a general practice, this is in many ways an extremely worthwhile venture. Not only is a personal relationship formed with the geriatrician who will be at the centre of attempts to solve many problems that the practitioner will experience with the elderly, but it will also enable him to gain an insight into the workings and facilities of the geriatric service to which he will be able to refer his patients.

SOCIAL SERVICES

Social workers

Social workers do not deal with all social problems. If an old person's principal problem is to do with her housing or income or is one of isolation and loneliness social workers are well equipped and willing to give good advice about the steps which the old person and her supporters could take to alleviate the problem, but a social worker would usually not wish to become directly involved in such problems. One of the responsibilities of a social services department is to act as an advice centre to the community it serves and it is the social workers who give advice on housing, heating, or income problems if a member of the public phones or calls, but advice and information on practical problems can also be obtained from a Housing Aid Centre or a Citizen's Advice Bureau or from the local office of Age Concern.

The second type of task performed by social workers is that they are responsible for the allocation of some of the resources of the social services department in which they work, notably places in old peoples' homes. This aspect of their work is not simply a type of hotel management, of looking for suitable vacant rooms for old people who refer, or are referred, for residential care. They have to assess the social needs of the person, decide whether or not admission to an institution is the most appropriate means of meeting their needs and then to compare that individual's need with the needs of all the other people deemed to need admission so that the available place can be allocated to the person in greatest need.

It is in the assessment of the social need that the skills of the Social Worker are most clearly demonstrated. She has to be able to discern and assess the significance not only of the practical problems which are apparently the sole reason why the elder is deemed to be in need of care but also of the beliefs, attitudes, and feelings of other people which are often as important as the practical problems in leading to the referral. The task is often made more difficult because in many families the relevant beliefs, attitudes, and emotions have never been expressed, indeed the old person and her supporters may have tried to conceal them from the professionals and even from one another. To what degree is a daughter's inability to support her mother due to unexpressed feelings of anger and resentment resulting from her mother's domination? Is the old person's wish to go into a home the result of feelings of guilt about the effect she thinks she is having on her son's marriage? It is this type of question which the social worker will ask and try to answer by helping all those involved to talk frankly about their feelings and motives although this approach may cause pain and distress. Of course assessment is not the sole objective of intervention; it is only the first step. The social worker will try to solve or alleviate the practical problems, try to help the old person and her supporters to modify or change their beliefs, attitudes, and feelings, in the hope that the old person will be able to continue to live at home.

The types of case which are referred to social workers by general practitioners are those in which it is thought that residential care is required and those in which it is thought that unspoken family tensions and pressures are making a significant contribution to the problems of the old person and her supporters. There is an obvious overlap between the functions of the general practitioner, the social worker, the psychiatrist, and the health visitor. All are trained to undertake this type of family therapy and the use which a general practitioner makes of these professionals will be influenced by many factors, notably his own interest in, and aptitude for, family problems, the degree of interest the health visitor has in this type of work, and his relationship with the local social work team and psychiatrist. Where the general practitioner thinks that residential care is appropriate for one of his elderly patients he will, of course, have to refer her to the social services department for assessment by a social worker no matter how well he knows, or thinks he knows, her needs.

It is essential to remember that social workers also have the right of referral to a general practitioner and if an old person has been referred to the social services department for residential care without the general practitioner's knowledge, as often happens, it is essential for local social workers to be able to discuss the referral with person's general practitioner. If the person is said to have deteriorated and if she has not seen her general practitioner in the recent past a medical review is indicated as part of the complete review of the elder's needs. Even if the general practitioner has seen the old person recently and if he is satisfied that nothing more can be done to reduce her disability it is almost always helpful for doctor and social worker to discuss the old person's needs.

Social work audit—a teaching aid for trainees

The trainer can help the trainee who has not worked in a department of geriatric medicine to learn about social work with elderly people by encouraging him to carry out a simple audit. Five referrals can be considered and the following questions asked.

1. What was the reason for the referral?
2. Did the health visitor and district nurse agree with the reason for referral?
3. What was the outcome of referral?
4. Was referral to the social services appropriate?
5. Did the social worker involved feel that she had been adequately informed by the primary care team?

In addition, it is also useful for the trainee to review the case notes of three people aged over eighty who are living alone and of another three who are living with families and to discuss with the social worker the following questions:

1. What are this person's principal social problems?
2. What are the problems of their supporters?
3. Would referral to the social services department or to any other agency be appropriate?

Home helps and organizers

The job of the home help is to help disabled elderly people to live at home. They do this by helping them with their housework and with food preparation, at least that is the physical component of their work, but in many cases it is the psychological help and support which is just as important as, or even more important than, the practical help.

OTHER HOSPITAL SERVICES

Although geriatric hospital services are of central importance in the care of older people other hospital specialties are also involved.

Community hospitals

It is now generally accepted that one of the major mistakes that was made in the evolution of the NHS was the closure of many small cottage hospitals: the 'economics of scale' argument held sway until the argument that 'small is beautiful' became fashionable and it was recognized that both large *and* small hospitals were needed. However, the need to define an operational policy for the small hospital was also recognized and this led to the development of the concept of the community hospital. Community hospitals are either cottage hospitals which have adopted a certain operational policy or, less commonly, they are purpose built.

The community hospital offers older patients a number of services.

> Emergency admissions for problems which cannot be managed at home but which do not need the services of the District General Hospital.
> Day hospital care.
> Rehabilitation.
> Intermittent admissions.
> Post-operative care.
> Long-stay care.

At present the great majority of community hospitals are in small towns, being cottage hospitals that escaped the scalpel during the era of closures, but there are experiments in the provision of community hospital care in the cities. The problems of organization of city community hospitals are much greater because more GPs have to be involved but these difficulties are not insuperable and an increasing proportion of GPs may be able to have access to hospital beds in the years to come.

Orthopaedic services

The elderly are commonly admitted to orthopaedic wards, both as accident and emergency cases and for elective operations.

Fractured neck of femur is a common disorder because the elderly fall more often and because their bones are thinner. Often the consequences of the fracture – the admission to hospital, the blood loss, the general anaesthetic, the metabolic response to trauma, and the immobility – are such that the person's ability to function is significantly and permanently reduced. The result of this is that the old person is forced to change her status, e.g. by requiring admission to an old people's home on discharge from hospital although she was living in her own home before.

In contrast, the old person who has an elective hip replacement may enjoy a significant improvement in her functional ability. More than half the people who have an elective hip replacement are over the age of 65 and this service, like pacemaker insertion, is a good example of the way in which 'high technology medicine' improves the quality of life of those older people who receive it.

Specialist hospital services

In addition to these two types of service almost every other specialist service provides care for the elderly. Obstetrics and paediatrics are obvious exceptions but in all other branches of the hospital services the elderly are an important group of patients, and all who work in hospital services need to be aware of the biological effects of aging and the influence these have on disease and on recovery, and to be sensitive to the ways in which the beliefs and attitudes of older patients influence presentation, compliance, and outcome.

Psychiatric hospitals

Although this book is not concerned primarily with psychiatric problems it would be inappropriate to review the hospital services for older people without emphasizing the part of the service with which GPs most often find difficulty – the psychiatric sector. The population of older people has been increasing just as the size of the psychiatric sector has been in decline and although older patients have taken an increasing proportion of the beds the psychogeriatric services have not developed sufficiently quickly to meet the needs of the elderly with mental disorders. No matter how willing the consultant may be he cannot admit a patient unless there are nurses to care for them. Beds are not in shortage; it is staffed beds that are lacking.

Residential care

Part III of the 1948 National Assistance Act stated that it 'shall be the duty of every local authority . . . to provide residential accommodation for persons who by reason of age, infirmity or any other circumstance are in need of care and attention which is not otherwise available to them'. This is the reason why local authority residential accommodation is often known as 'Part III' but neither Part II nor Part IV of the Act had anything to do with residential care, although the latter is sometimes used as a euphemism for heaven when discussing a patient's prospects in her presence. Sheltered housing is sometimes known as Category 2 housing. This is a reference to a circular which had nothing to do with the National Assistance Act although some people refer to sheltered housing as 'Part 2'.

The need for permanent care

An old person's need for permanent admission to Part III is determined by two factors: firstly by the effects of her 'age, infirmity or any other circumstances' and secondly by the amount and type of domiciliary care which is 'otherwise available' as an alternative to admission.

The degree of disability or infirmity is obviously of importance as 'age' *per se* is obviously irrelevant. It is the responsibility of the patient's General Practitioner to ensure that her disability is as little as it can be but he also has to remember that 'other circumstances' may be the cause of the person's need for 'care and attention'. Three other circumstances always have to be taken into account:

1. The physical environment as this has an important bearing on the degree to which the disabled person is handicapped (see p. 160).

2. The person's personality because some people are better motivated than others and are less likely to become dependent. In addition, some are much more pleasant and rewarding than others thus inspiring a much greater degree of loyalty and commitment in their supporters who are willing to help them for much longer than they would be willing to help someone who is unrewarding and ungrateful.

3. The attitudes of other people, for if an old person is repeatedly told 'you

can't manage and you would be better off in a home' she may come to believe it herself.

It is, however, the second factor – the amount of 'care and attention . . . otherwise available' – which is of even greater importance. An old person's need for residential care is usually justified in terms of her disability and dependence but it is the level of domiciliary service which is of crucial importance. The more help available at home the longer will an old person be able to live there and the later will be a 'need' for a residential care defined.

When an old person is referred to the general practitioner as being 'in need of care', and referrals usually come from third parties and not from old people themselves, the doctor should ask five questions:

Question	Action
1. Could her disability be reduced by improving diagnosis, treatment, or compliance, or by physiotherapy? (See p. 162)	Review clinical status with referral to a consultant in geriatric medicine if in any doubt. A domiciliary consultation is often very useful in this situation. Ask for the advice of a physiotherapist if direct referral is possible and if unsatisfied that diagnosis and treatment are appropriate and do not need a second medical opinion.
2. Could her handicap be reduced by modifying her environment?	Ask the advice of a domiciliary occupational therapist.
3. Could her motivation be improved to reduce her dependance on other people?	Review the case with other professionals who know the old person.
4. Could the attitudes of other people be more constructive and helpful?	Discuss the problem with all those whose attitudes and opinions you feel to be relevant. At some point a discussion which brings together everyone who has an interest should be arranged. It may be that the health visitor or a social worker would be more effective and if referral has been made to a social services department the social workers will take this approach. The attitudes of other people can be most easily modified by relieving guilt and providing practical help, for example by relieving a family by a series of short-term admissions or by day care.
5. How much help is the old person receiving in her own home?	Request more help from the district nurse, and if necessary the nursing officer, and the home help organizer. We believe that it is not unreasonable to request two visits a day from the domiciliary nursing service on every days of the week and two visits from a home help on weekdays with one visit on Saturdays and Sundays supplemented by voluntary help before a person who wishes to remain in her own home is said to be in need of residential accommodation. In addition, day care and intermittent admissions to an old people's home or hospital should also be considered.

Even if the old person herself says that she wishes to go to live in a home it is worth while reviewing her case in this way because she may change her mind when an alternative is offered to her.

Day care

Day care at an old people's home can be helpful in a number of situations of which five are common:

1. To relieve the effects of isolation.
2. To allow the old person to try the home so that she may decide whether or not she would like to be admitted as a permanent resident.
3. As a means of allowing the staff of the home to see if they can cope with her.
4. To introduce the old person to the home, its residents, and its staff once she has definitely decided that she would like to leave her own home.
5. To provide temporary relief for the old person's relatives and professional supporters.

Some old people are reluctant to go to day care. The reason for this may be that the old person has been alone for so long that she is nervous of meeting other people. In addition, she may be ashamed of her appearance. This attitude can usually be changed if the old person is helped to buy new clothes and have her hair washed and set and if she can be accompanied by someone whom she trusts for the first visit or two. Refusal may be due to difficulty with dressing and it may be necessary for the old person to be helped to dress before the transport comes to collect her.

The old person may refuse to go because she suspects that the suggestion of day care is only a ruse and that she will be kept in the home. The only way to overcome this reason is to assure the old person that she is not being deceived and to use the person she trusts most, who may be the Home Help, to convince her that she is not being tricked out of her home. Finally, the old person may refuse simply because she does not wish to go and does not see how she will benefit from day care. Not infrequently this reason for refusal is encountered when the reason for day care is not to benefit the old person but to relieve other people, and unless the old person is told honestly the real reason why day care is being suggested, preferably by the person who will benefit, and helped to see that it is in her interests to offer relief to her supporters, it is entirely reasonable of her to refuse.

Intermittent admissions

It is always possible to arrange an admission of limited duration to allow relatives to go on holiday, for example for two weeks in the summer, but relatives must be encouraged to book early. In addition the practice of offering a regular series of short admissions is increasing, the old person being offered two weeks in every eight weeks or some other similar pattern. The situations in which this type of admission are helpful, and the reasons why old people sometimes refuse to enter a home for a short spell, are the same as those discussed in the section on day care.

It is not uncommon for the staff of the home to report in the week following admission that the old person is not so fit as they were led to believe and this is of particular significance if the old person's fitness for permanent residence is being tested by the staff. There are many possible reasons for this but one which is of particular importance is the relocation effect because it can be minimised by careful preparation.

The relocation effect

This is the name given to the changes which occur when a person moves from one environment to another. The changes may be beneficial as, for example, when an old person's physical and mental state improves following a move to sheltered housing. This is sometimes termed a positive relocation effect to distinguish it from a negative or harmful relocation effect. Negative effects take many forms. Confusion may increase, behaviour problems may develop, and the old person's condition may deteriorate; a move may even cause the death of the old person.

The nature and degree of the reaction of an old person to environmental change are functions of many factors which can be grouped into three main types, each of which can be modified by those who are helping the old person make the change.

The individual's personality and attitudes are obviously important. Some people are more adaptable than others and it is obviously difficult to change basic personality traits, but there is one factor which can be influenced – the willingness of the person to move. Those people who are unwilling to move are more likely to be adversely affected by a move than those who move willingly. A person may be unwilling to move not only because she has happy memories associated with her home but also because she feels that she has not been properly consulted about the decision, or that more could be done to keep her in her own home or that she is the victim of a conspiracy. The general practitioner cannot, of course, dispel the happy associations which her home has for her but he can try to ensure that everything possible has been tried before permanent care is suggested, the old person is given every opportunity to be involved in the plans for her future, and that the matter is conducted as openly and honestly as possible. If one of the reasons why the old person has to go to live in a home is that the relatives with whom she lives need relief it is better that this is admitted openly by the relatives, even though that admission may cause both them and the old person distress, than for everyone to say to the old person that it is for her own good that she needs to be in a home.

The second important factor is the style of the transition from home to institution; the more abrupt the transition the greater the risk of a negative relocation effect. In emergencies an abrupt transition is necessary but where a move is planned it is possible to allow the person to adapt to her new environment and to the idea of living there. Day care, followed by admissions of short duration, are very helpful and it is a reasonable rule to state that no-one should go to live permanently in a home without having had the opportunity of living in that home for at least two weeks, preferably much longer. When the move is finally made it is important that the elder should take as much of her home with her as possible but even more important is that she be given adequate support during the transitional period. The provision of help and support during this time is one of the main contributions which a General Practitioner can make to the wellbeing of an elderly person who is leaving her home. In addition it is very supportive to the old person, and often to the staff of the home also, if he can keep her on his list for a few months after admission, and be prepared to travel some distance to visit her, even though the distance is so great that she will ultimately have to transfer to another list. Not only does this reduce the number of changes the elder must make but it is easier for the doctor who has known a person for some years to assess the extent and significance of the effects of relocation than it is for a doctor who has only known her since she moved. Both the staff and the new doctor may assume that she has always been as disabled as she appears in the early weeks following the move and miss the fact that she has deteriorated because of the move.

The third type of factor, over which the doctor has least influence, is that which relates to the institution to which the old person moves. Negative relocation effects are less common, and less severe if they should occur, the more loving, warm, and relaxed the institution. It is obviously difficult for a general practitioner to influence the nature of the home to which his patient is going to move but he can make one important contribution. He can give the home confidence that if the old person becomes ill or more disabled he will do all he can to help and support them. The staff of residential homes face an extremely difficult job with many demands made of them by residents, relatives, and other professionals. The more help they receive the more energy will they have to devote to the residents. The general practitioner who encourages staff to consult him, who tries to visit the home regularly and does not only visit to deal with problems, who offers to help with in-service training, who introduces new nursing staff to the homes, and who tries to offer his skills and experience to the home can contribute to the health and wellbeing of the home and this will help all the residents including the new resident.

Private and voluntary homes

Voluntary homes are run by voluntary organizations such as the Methodist Church and the Salvation Army. Private homes are usually run by the proprietor. Some homes are designated as old people's homes and registered with the social services department, others are registered with the health authority as nursing homes, but there is little practical difference between the two.

Elderly people and their relatives should be advised to think of a private or voluntary home when:

1. The old person wishes to move from one part of the country to another; most local authorities are so hard pressed that they can only give a low priority to elderly people who wish to move nearer relatives. However, private and voluntary homes are not constrained in this way. The old person and her relatives should also be told to consider a move to sheltered housing, provided by a housing association (see p. 186) in these circumstances.

2. The old person has specific religious needs; there are homes for Catholics, Jews, and Methodists.

3. The old person is eligible for a particular voluntary home or type of home, such as the Chelsea Hospital or the Masonic homes.

4. The old person is considered unfit for Part III but too fit for hospital.

5. The old person wishes a higher standard of accommodation than that offered by the local authority; remember, however, that some private and voluntary homes have lower standards than local authority homes.

In these circumstances an old person and her relatives can be advised to take the following steps:

1. To write asking the social services department for a list of registered old people's homes and if there is someone who can advise them on their relative merits.

2. To write to the district medical officer asking for a list of registered nursing homes and if there is someone who can give advice on their merits.

3. To ask for help from GRACE – Mrs Gould's Residential Advisory Centre for the Elderly (Leigh Comer, Leigh Hill Road, Cobham, Surrey) and Counsel and Care for the Elderly (131 Middlesex Street, London E1 7JF) which both act as advisory services. The Registered Nursing Homes Association (7-7A Station Road, Finchley, London N3 2SB) also provides information.

4. Consult the *Charities Digest* which lists many of the voluntary homes.

The cost for private and voluntary homes is about the same as the cost of local authority care but the old person is entitled to her pension and to an Attendance Allowance when a resident and these benefits reduce the weekly charge considerably.

6 Are older patients different?

Older patients obviously have more disease than younger patients but does that justify a whole book devoted to their problems? Is the challenge for general practice not simply that there will be more old people and that these old people have more diseases? We believe that there are important differences and that the approach to older patients has to be different from the approach to younger people. In part this is due to the fact that the presentation and the natural history of disease in old age and the response to treatment can also differ, but there are also important social and cultural differences which have a bearing on aspects of medicine such as self-referral, referral by others and compliance, and it is these differences which we wish to consider in this chapter.

HEALTH BELIEFS AND ATTITUDES

Disease, disability, and handicap are all more common among older people and the general level of satisfaction with health is therefore lower among older people than among younger people (Fig. 6.1).

Many who are dissatisfied obviously seek help from their general practitioner but some who are dissatisfied do not, because they believe that it would be a waste of time. In addition, some of the people who are satisfied, and who therefore do not make demands on their general practitioner, are suffering from treatable disorders. Both these factors influence demand and are the consequences of certain beliefs and attitudes (Becker 1971).

'It's my age'

Many old people do not appreciate the distinction between disease and aging and assume that every problem is due to 'old age'. Because it is widely known that there is no cure for old age, no elixir of life, the old person either accepts it philosophically – 'What else can you expect at my age, other people are worse off' or becomes depressed or bitter and dissatisfied but does not seek help – 'What's the use, the doctors are busy and they should help those they can cure'.

This confusion between the effects of normal aging and the effects of disease is apparently more common for certain signs and symptoms. There are certain disorders in which the majority of those affected are known and others in which only a minority are known (Figs. 6.2 and 6.3).

As Professor Williamson emphasizes, the fact that some disabilities are less likely to be known to the person's doctor than others is not simply a matter of sociological interest, it is of vital clinical importance.

Health beliefs and attitudes 113

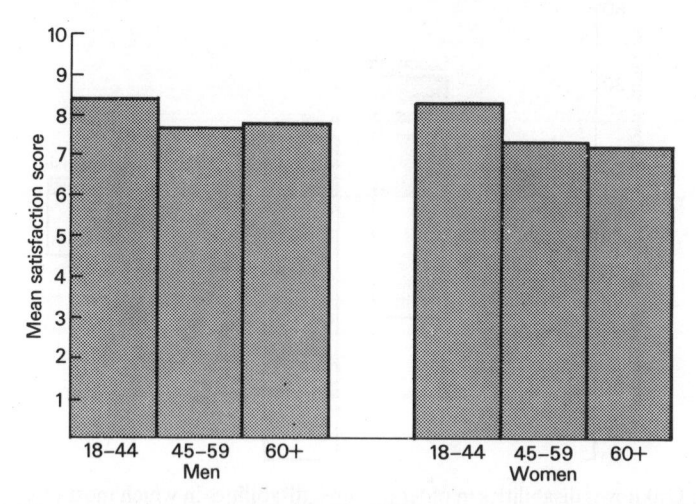

Fig. 6.1. Mean satisfaction scores for health. (SSRC survey of 1900 people, reported in *Profiles of the elderly,* Vol. 1. Age Concern, London (1977).)

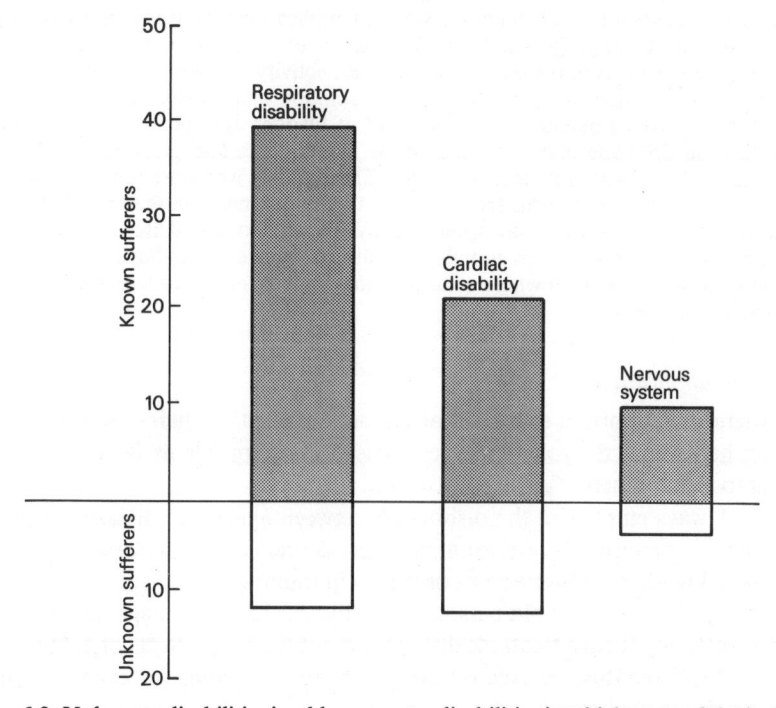

Fig. 6.2. Unknown disabilities in older persons: disabilities in which most of the iceberg is above water (practitioner's awareness is relatively high). (Williamson 1981.)

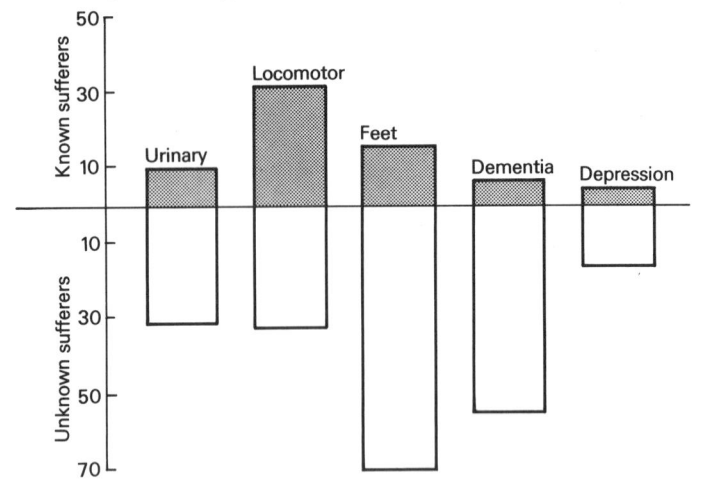

Fig. 6.3. Unknown disabilities in older persons: disabilities in which most of the iceberg is submerged (practitioner's awareness is low). (Williamson 1981.)

It is interesting to note that these largely known disabilities are of great importance for the affected individual and possess special implications. Thus locomotor disabilities are painful and progressive and they lead to restriction of mobility. Hence they may readily lead to impoverishment of social activity, difficulty in shopping and hence carry the danger of producig social isolation and loneliness and eventually apathy and risk of malnutrition. The onset of bladder dysfunction, in males post-micturition dribbling and in females stress incontinence and precipitancy, lead to considerable distress and embarrassment. The old lady who dare not allow herself to be more than a few yards from a toilet, or the old man whose underclothes are frequently wet with urine, may often react by limitation of social life and consequent dangers of isolation and low morale. Perhaps the greatest risk, however, is for the elderly dementing patient whose condition goes undetected until a late stage. (Williamson 1981).

Practical implications

It is therefore important to try to learn about a patient's beliefs – most easily by asking her 'What do you think the cause of your problems is' and then by trying to modify them.

   Always emphasize the distinction between aging and disease whenever there is opportunity, for example at pre-retirement lectures and in talks to social workers or home helps or priests in training.

   Emphasize to the old person whose disease has been diagnosed that she is suffering from a treatable disease and not from the effects of aging.

   Reinforce this message on every possible occasion, for example when reviewing medication.

   Educate relatives about the difference between aging and disease and ask them to keep reminding their elder of the distinction.

'It's God's Will'

Some old people believe that they are affected by disease because it is 'God's Will', some believe that God has caused or 'sent' the disease; others, more commonly, that He has let it happen. It is important to appreciate that the person who holds this view does not reject scientific explanations of disease causation, for example accepting a general practitioner's explanation of the reasons why joints are painful and stiff, and that there is a disease called rheumatoid arthritis caused by a process which is not fully understood. A religious person therefore is prepared to accept that disease has a cause but may ask why it is that he or she should be suffering from rheumatoid arthritis when other people do not have the disease. 'Why me? Why am I suffering?'

This type of fatalistic view is particularly influential among elderly Moslems who believe in the Will of Allah and among strict Presbyterians who may add 'God willing', or 'DV' as a conditional clause when discussing the possible outcome of some procedure such as an operation, but it is common among all faiths. Fortunately most people who believe that this is the reason they are suffering also believe that antibiotics, anaesthetics, the skills of doctors, and all the other benefits of modern medicine are other manifestations of God's Will so that it is uncommon for an old person to refuse treatment because she believes that it is wrong or pointless to try to influence God's Will. Some elders are, however, more fatalistic than others, and prayer, with the support of a priest, can help some old people. A priest can also be useful in convincing an elder that it is possible for her condition to improve and in increasing her faith in the treatment offered, both of which should improve compliance.

Another problem resulting from this type of religious belief is the suffering which can be caused by unresolved religious conflicts. Some old people believe that their disease is a punishment for some transgression. A person with this believe feels perplexed initially because he believes that he has led a good life. He then thinks back, looking for a reason for his punishment, and because it is always possible to find possible reasons why one should be punished, some minor sexual pecadillo or some act of dishonesty, he may begin to brood about his sins and become emotionally disturbed. If he accepts that his punishment is just he will probably be depressed and may be poorly motivated to get better because he believes that he deserves to suffer. If, on the other hand, he thinks that his suffering is undeserved, he may feel angry or resentful – 'Why me, why am I suffering, what have I done to deserve this?' – and this type of attitude may reduce the efficacy of treatment which has been prescribed for the relief of symptoms, because pain and other types of discomfort are much more difficult to control with drugs if the person is angry or resentful about his suffering than if he is tranquil and relatively detached.

Practical implications

The religious dimension should always be remembered when assessing an old person. A question such as 'Do you ever wonder why you are suffering in this way when others are spared?' may be a useful opening. The person may answer that it is 'just bad luck' or 'just one of those things', suggesting that she believes that the incidence of disease is randomly distributed, or they may reply in religious terms. If she does it is easy to suggest that she might like to speak to a priest if she is not in regular contact with one. This is, however, a topic which some elders will not wish to discuss and may be inappropriate unless there is a good relationship between doctor and patient.

The general practitioner should be prepared to reveal his own views on religion and suffering if he opens up this line of discussion and if he believes in the existence of God should be prepared to discuss why God lets evil and suffering exist. If it is thought inappropriate to raise this topic directly the old person can be asked if she used to attend church in the context of discussing her social isolation, for example by saying 'Perhaps we could arrange for you to get out of the house a bit more, to go where you used to go. Did you go to church regularly?' If the person says that she did but that she is no longer able to attend it is appropriate to ask for the help of the priest either to visit her or, better, to see if he can arrange for transport to take her to worship with other people regularly again. By involving the priest on the pretext of reducing her social isolation the old person is offered the opportunity of discussing her suffering with someone who may help her appreciate the meaning of her suffering and relieve any feelings of guilt.

Close links between local priests and the primary care team are important.

'I can't do it; it'll never work'

Older people are, in general, more pessimistic than younger people and there are two reasons for this. Firstly, their generation has been disappointed so often that many of its members have become disillusioned. 'It Will All Be Over By Christmas', 'Homes Fit For Heroes', 'The War to End All Wars', 'Peace In Our Time' – these and many other promises have been made but not kept. Members of this generation have had their hopes dashed so often that they have learned to be cautious to preclude disappointment (Gray and Wilcock 1981; Blythe 1979).

The second reason some older people are pessimistic is because of their experience while becoming disabled. Progressive disability is a succession of failures. At first the person becomes unable to complete a round of golf, then even a few holes become impossible, then he finds it impossible to reach his local pub or shops, then the front gate becomes too far for him to reach and finally he may fail to reach the toilet because he cannot climb the stairs. The pessimism which results from increasing disability may be compounded by the failure of professionals to produce what they promise. Disabled people are commonly disappointed by professionals who raise their hopes about rehousing, or the provision of a telephone, or day care, or a number of other services without delivering the goods. As a result of these many disappointments an old person may become very pessimistic and refuse to consider the possibility of improving his condition or circumstances as a means of precluding yet another disappointment.

Practical implications

The best means of overcoming pessimism is success; success by the old person in doing something for herself, and professional success in achieving what was promised. Faced with a multitude of problems the old person may be overwhelmed by the size and scale of her problems and too pessimistic to try to overcome them. To overcome this try to identify one or two small soluble problems and set one or two short-term and achievable goals. When these are achieved new goals can be set and other small problems solved.

'I've known worse'

Some older patients are satisfied because their present position is not too bad in comparison with the problems they have had to face.

> Mr S. was an Old Contemptible. Disabled by a stroke and suffering from bronchitis he lived in a large, old council dwelling and the room which he used as a bedroom was very damp. His doctor and social worker attempted to obtain sufficient funds to install a gas fire in his bedroom without success. They broke the news to him somewhat hesitantly, fearing that he would feel disappointed. He took the news without a qualm and tried to reassure the disappointed professionals by saying 'Don't worry: sixty years ago today I was up to my waist in mud and water'.

It is not uncommon for an old person's situation to be defined as 'a problem' by younger relatives or professionals when the old person herself perceives no cause for dissatisfaction. The heating and financial difficulties of elderly people are often severe, but if an old person suffered even more severely in the nineteen-twenties and thirties they may be of little significance to her. The old woman who had to feed her young family in the twenties during the long years when her husband was unemployed may regard herself as 'well off' although she is impoverished by the standards of her professional helpers. A woman who has had to choose which child should have the only egg or who has had to try to disguise from her husband the fact that she is hungry so that he may eat, as many an older woman has had to do, may find her present financial problems comparatively easy to bear.

The satisfaction of elderly people with the services they are given is due to the same influences and to the fact that older people were brought up in a time in which the individual had fewer rights than people now enjoy. As a result of this many do not think of the services they are offered as their right and are more grateful than younger people, most of whom perceive health and social services as their right.

One other factor must be taken into account when considering an old person's satisfaction – fatigue. Many disabled old people find the prospect of the effort which they believe will be necessary to effect a change so daunting that they prefer not to make the effort. It is not that such people are intellectually incapable of change but they are tired. They may have worked hard for fifty or sixty years and the memories of this, together with the fatigue which results from the effort which disabled people have to expend to perform simple tasks, encourage their faith in the *status quo*. This attitude was clearly enunciated by J. B. Priestley in his autobiography *'Instead of the Trees'* when he wrote:

> Because I am old, almost everything demands both effort and patience. Nothing runs itself. What – even getting dressed or going to bed? Certainly. They are both workouts. I do not say tremendous efforts are involved, but there are no easy routines here, nothing accomplished while thinking about something else. I can have a little wrestling match just getting into a pair of trousers. Just coping with the mere arrangements of ordinary living, there must continually be an exercise of will. To get by from nine in the morning until midnight I use enough willpower to command an army corps.

Practical implications

It is difficult to change this attitude except by pointing out that although things 'could be worse' that they could also be better, but it has to be remembered that if an old person is satisfied with her lot it may be unethical to make her dissatisfied, with the objective of motivating her to accept change.

'I don't want any help, thank you'

Some people refuse help not because they are satisfied with their position but because they are frightened of what 'help' may imply. The over-riding fear is that of institutionalization, of being 'put in a home', and an old person who has this fear may try to deceive the doctor who is trying to assess her. Consider what may pass through the mind of an old person who is asked 'Can you do your housework by yourself?', or 'Are you able to bathe yourself?'. If she is unable to do so the old person has to decide whether or not it will be prudent to reveal her difficulties. It would seem obvious that she should, so that her need for help can be identified but some old people feel that to answer such questions in the affirmative may lead not to domiciliary help but to the suggestion, followed by powerful persuasion, that she 'would be better off in a home'. Similarly, some old people are afraid that to answer 'yes' to the question 'Are you lonely?' may also lead to the suggestion that she 'would be better off in a home'.

Old people, therefore, not infrequently deceive those who come to help them. They may exaggerate their abilities and minimize their disabilities or tell lies, giving the answers which they believe will satisfy their interviewers that they are able to continue living at home.

Practical implications

Of all the professionals the general practitioner is usually trusted more than any other but even if there is a relationship in which mutual trust is a strong feature the old person may be suspicious and guarded when the doctor comes to visit her in a crisis at the request of anxious relatives, who want the doctor to 'persuade' her to agree to something 'for her own good' or to 'make her see sense' or to make her see 'the reality of the situation'. To reassure the old person can be difficult but the following ideas may be helpful.

An explicit statement such as 'I'm here to help you stay on in your own home if that's what you want to do' made early in the interview can be very reassuring. The importance of touching, by holding hands, as a means of reassurance should not be underestimated and an introductory handshake can be sustained for this purpose.

The old person should be asked if she feels that any problems are particularly troublesome and asked what she thinks would be the best solution in each problem.

The word 'help' is vague and may therefore be threatening: 'We want to help you' may be taken to mean 'We want you to go into a home'.

Section 47

'Section 47', as it is known among doctors and social workers, concerns persons who:

(a) are suffering from grave chronic disease or, being aged, infirm or physically incapacitated, are living in insanitary conditions, and

(b) are unable to devote to themselves, and are not receiving from other persons, proper care and attention.

It lays down that they may be removed from their homes if it is in their 'interest', or if it is necessary to prevent 'injury to the health of, or serious nuisance to, other persons'. The power to approach a magistrate for a removal order was given to the Medical Officer of Health in 1948, and is now vested in the Medical Officer for Environmental Health to the District Council in which the elder lives, because, rather surprisingly, it was given to district councils in 1974 along with environmental responsibilities rather than to the authorities responsible for health or social services. The Medical Officer for Environmental Health, a community physician, has to apply to a court or a magistrate, giving seven days' notice of the intended removal. If an order is issued, the person can be detained for three months in 'a suitable hospital or other place' (Gray 1980).

The National Assistance (Amendment) Act 1951 allows for immediate removal but the Medical Officer for Environmental Health must include the recommendation of another doctor, usually the person's General Practitioner, that the person be removed without delay, but an order for immediate removal allows the person's detention for no more than three weeks. This Amendment Act was introduced as a Private Member's Bill, with Government support, by the late Sir Alfred Broughton, a doctor, who was Member for Batley and Morley. His constituents had been shocked by the death of a lady who had lain on the floor of her house, refusing all offers of help, watched by neighbours and officials, while the seven statutory days' notice expired, because she developed a pressure sore and tetanus during this period.

The person does not need to be mentally ill for the powers to be invoked but in a high proportion of the cases in which it has been used the elderly person is not completely competent, either due to a mild degree of dementia or to a toxic confusional state or a combination of both. It is very difficult to generalize about the types of case in which Section 47 would be appropriate because the interpretation of the Act is left to the discretion of the Community Physician. The types of problem in which Section 47 might be appropriate are:

    Where a person has a treatable condition, such as a fractured femur, provided that treatment can only be given in hospital.

    Where the person was willing to seek and accept treatment until recently and has only recently begun to refuse offers of help.

    The types of problem for which Section 47 is inappropriate are:

    Where the main problem is the accumulation of dirt and refuse, blocked drains, rats and mice: the Environmental Health officer has powers to deal with such problems, using the Public Health Acts.

    Where the person has been a recluse and refused help for years or decades.

If the person only requires more care than she can be given in her own home and not a type of treatment which can only be given in hospital: it is unreasonable to consider removing a person who does not need specialzed treatment until she has gone beyond the limits of care which can be given by two district nurse and two home help visits a day.

If the old person is either 'at risk' or is putting other people at risk.

These powers are seldom used but it is occasionally more honest and less traumatic to use them than to continue sustained efforts to 'persuade' the old person to agree to go to hospital to such an extent that she finally gives in and complies with the wishes of others simply to gain respite from their vehement arguments.

BELIEFS AND ATTITUDES OF OTHER PEOPLE
(Gray and Wilcock 1981b)

Underestimation

Many people believe that all people over the age of sixty-five – all 'the elderly' – are of declining physical capacity and intelligence and that they are unable to change, learn, or improve, and some even believe that all old people are 'dementing'. This prejudice is sometimes called ageism and it leads to an underestimation of the abilities of older people and an underestimation of the potential for treatment and rehabilitation.

The friends and relatives of elderly people may accept physical changes such as breathlessness, deafness, or incontinence as being due to 'old age' and therefore not seek professional help. Underestimation can also cause problems with compliance. If relatives are to be involved in supervising medication they have to be as carefully educated about the difference between disease and aging as the elderly person. If they are to be involved in a programme of rehabilitation, for example in reinforcing the physiotherapist's advice, they have to be convinced that the old person will be able to learn to be independent again.

Ageism can cause and aggravate mental disorder. Frequently the relatives, friends, and professional helpers of elderly people agree with them whatever they say. If the old person makes a mistake in the days of the week, or her address, or some other factual detail, they say 'yes, yes', or 'oh really?' or they utter some other agreeable platitude. This can be very frustrating, depressing, and confusing. We all depend on other people correcting our mistakes to avoid confusion and old people have a right to be disagreed with even when they suffer from dementia.

Ageism can also cause and aggravate behaviour disorders. Often behaviour problems have developed because no-one has told the old person that his behaviour is upsetting other people. Everyone depends upon the checks and corrections of other people to limit his or her behaviour and old people have a right to be checked and corrected like younger people.

Useful advice for old people and their relatives

Communicating with old people

If some physical or mental change develops over a short period of time, for example a few weeks or a few months, or if a change can be noticed to have occurred since some particular date, for example 'since Christmas' or 'since we visited at Easter' the advice of the doctor, district nurse, or health visitor should be sought to ensure that it is not a sign of a treatable disease.

Don't make too many allowances because of a person's age. Old people are different because they have had different experiences. Their attitude and outlook differs from yours in some respects. Remember that when speaking to them but try to converse with the old person as you would talk to someone aged thirty-five. If you would correct or disagree with a thirty-five year old person correct or disagree with the old person.

If the old person keeps making the same mistakes, for example, by asking the same question again and again, change the subject.

If she becomes very distressed by your disagreement or correction be prepared to give in but remember that elderly people are as entitled to have a good argument as younger people.

Be careful of disagreeing with an old person who believes that her husband is still alive.

122 *Are older patients different?*

Practical implications

Supporters and untrained professional helpers, such as the nursing auxiliary, often need education. The points in the table on the previous page should be emphasized when speaking to relatives.

The fact that many children have even greater reluctance to disagree with or correct their parents than professionals have should always be remembered and they may need more help in adopting an approach which is not agist (see p. 000).

Guilt

Doctors are often phoned by anxious neighbours and relatives. The reason for anxiety is guilt. The person who is anxious may be aware of the fact that he could do much more himself to help the old person if only he were to make more effort and he puts pressure on other people to 'do something' as a means of alleviating his guilt. It is this type of guilt which gives rise to what has been called the VR referral – the referral from the visiting relative on a Sunday evening, often made after he has returned to his own home.

The anxiety of other people may lead them to put pressure on the old person to agree to enter a home with the result that she may become depressed, or defensive, or even paranoid. Over-anxious relatives may make an old person afraid of the general practitioner by telling her that they have asked him to come to see her to 'make her see sense'. They may even have told her that the general practitioner will have her 'put away' if she does not agree to go. Over anxious people may refuse to help the old person in an attempt to force the professionals to act. They may also try to involve a number of different services, without telling any service that the others have been involved, playing off one against the other.

The general practitioner should, therefore, ask the referrer what his principal anxieties are about the old person and what the anxieties of other people are. Common anxieties are that the old person is at risk of malnutrition because she is not eating three meals a day, or at risk of setting fire to herself, or at risk of hypothermia, or at risk of falling. With such anxieties the person needs to be reassured that he will not be held responsible if the elder suffers in the way he fears, and it is helpful to state this explicitly even though the risk is small. If there is a real risk then steps should obviously be taken to reduce it and the person who is anxious should be involved in reducing the risk if at all possible. For example, if a relative is worried about malnutrition he can be asked to buy a flask and a sandwich box and told that if he prepares sandwiches and a hot flask every morning the old person will be adequately nourished without a cooked lunch.

Sometimes the cause of the anxiety is not revealed because the person is unaware of it or is ashamed of it. Relatives are often anxious that they are going to be asked to take their elder to live with them and should be explicitly reassured about this at the first interview. Some people are reluctant to admit that they are anxious about the risk to themselves or their families, usually a risk of fire or a gas explosion, preferring to say that it is the old person's wellbeing which is their main concern. However, they should be encouraged to admit their anxiety and told that it is reasonable for them to be concerned about their own safety.

Practical implications

Relatives who are doing as much as they can but who are still very anxious can be helped if the possible causes of anxiety are considered and discussed with them. It may be necessary to reassure the relatives by explicitly relieving them of a number of responsibilities which are common causes of guilt and over-protective anxiety. Relatives need to be reassured that:

> They are not going to be asked to take the old person to live with them.
> They will not be held responsible if something happens to the old person.
> The old person who wishes to live on at home has a right to be at risk.

Attitudes towards professional services

The expectations which relatives, neighbours, and friends have of health and social services are also determined by their beliefs and their attitudes, and their beliefs are often mistaken. Relatives may believe that any old person who is having difficulty in managing in her own home is entitled to go and live in an old people's home, or believe that it is part of a general practitioner's duty to visit their elder every month. If, however, their expectations are unrealistically great solely because of a mistaken belief it is usually fairly simple to modify them. It is much more difficult to influence expectations when they are the consequence of the relatives' hostile attitudes towards public servants.

Many people are hostile towards the health and social services and to those who work in them. Such people are of the opinion that because they pay rates and taxes they are justified in making any demands on services which they think necessary. This attitude is understandable because public services are paid for by rate and tax payers but if the person is also jealous of the professionals' secure, well-paid, superannuated jobs his demands may be stimulated as much by his desire to see some action by the public servicants, whom he believes to be over paid and underemployed, as by his concern for his elderly relative. This attitude is, understandably, commoner among people in insecure jobs at risk of bankruptcy, such as small businessmen and shopkeepers, or redundancy, for example people working in industry. Where the general practitioner is making a medical decision concerning treatment he is relatively immune from the pressure which this type of attitude can generate. however, in cases in which the family believe that the old person only requires 'caring for' as opposed to skilled treatment, they may apply considerable pressure on the general practitioner to admit the old person to hospital if she is not fit for an old people's home, or to persuade the old person to go into a home if she is reluctant to agree to do so.

Professional beliefs and attitudes

It is important to remember that professional training does not necessarily change these attitudes. In fact, they are reinforced by some teachers. It is, therefore, important to discuss these attitudes and beliefs with trainees and other professionals in training as well as with the relatives, neighbours, and friends of elderly people.

IMMOBILITY

As we have mentioned, immobility is one of the common handicaps in old age (see p. 45). Elderly patients find more difficulty in reaching the surgery than younger patients for three reasons:

1. Disabling disease is more common.
2. Car ownership is less common (Table 6.1).
3. They find it more difficult to use public transport than younger people (Fig. 6.4)

All in all, about two million elderly people find public transport dauntingly difficult. These mobility problems obviously limits the ability of the older person to initiate contact with the doctor, nurse, or health visitor. In addition, two other factors must be taken into account – isolation and telephone ownership.

Table 6.1. *Percentage in each age-group who drive and who have a car in the household*

	% who drive	% with car in household*
65–69	26.9	43.0
70–74	15.9	29.7
75–79	7.0	22.0
80–84	6.6	26.1
85 and over	1.4	24.8

*Including bedfast and housebound.
Hunt, A. (1978). *The elderly at home,* p. 111. HMSO, London.

Isolation

Old people live alone more frequently than younger people and therefore less frequently benefit from one particular type of consultation – the type which arises by chance when a doctor visits someone else in the house. This point was emphasized by Ann Cartwright and Robert Anderson in their 1977 study *General practice revisited,* for 43 per cent of the people in the study who were over 75 lived alone (Cartwright and Anderson 1981).

Lack of a telephone

Furthermore, those who are at greatest risk and in greatest need have the lowest rates of access to a phone. Only 35.4 per cent of elderly people who live alone and the same percentage of those who are over 85 years old have phones.

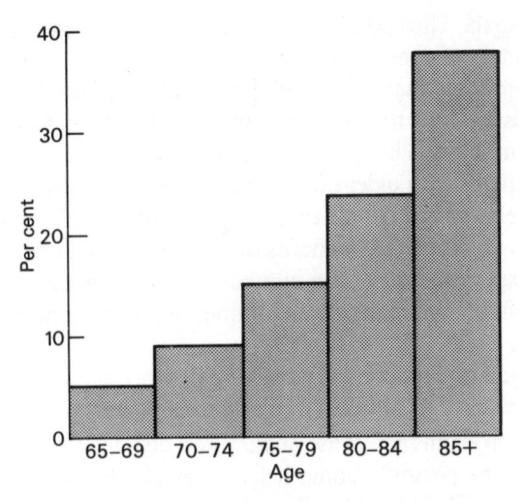

Fig. 6.4. Percentage either totally unable to use public transport or unable to do so without help. (From Hunt, A. (1978). *The elderly at home*, p. 74. HMSO, London.)

Table 6.2. *Telephone ownership*

Percentages	Households with an old person as head	Households with a young person as head
Having a phone in their own dwelling	39.3	72.1
Having a phone nearby, for example, in a hall or landing	1.9	0

From Hunt, A. (1978). *The elderly at home*, p. 53. HMSO, London.

Practical implications

Cartwright and Anderson reported a drop in home visiting since their earlier study of general practice in 1971. Half of those people aged over 75 who were interviewed said that they had not had any visit from a general practitioner in the last year and 11 per cent of this age group said that their doctor had never visited their home. There appears to have been no compensatory increase in surgery consultations, in fact the same trend can be seen (see p. 12), and neither does it seem that the increase in contacts made by health visitors and district nurses has been sufficient to make up for the decline in patient contact.

The implications are that any attempt to practice anticipatory care cannot rely solely on contacts initiated by patients, as is the case with preventive care for younger people. For example, the prevention of arterial disease by the detection and treatment of hypertension can be effectively done by 'case finding', that is, by taking the opportunity offered by any consultation to enquire about hypertension and other coronary side-factors. This approach is effective because the general practitioner will see 90 per cent of those on his list

126 *Are older patients different?*

in a five-year span. Thus 90 per cent coverage can be achieved without having to invite patients to a consultation or initiate contact in other ways. With older patients it is probable that at least 90 per cent also consult in a five-year span but five years is too long to wait in a population in which deterioration can take place quickly, mobility is limited, and expectations are low. To practice effective preventive medicine with older people the primary care team has therefore to be prepared to see more old people than initiate contact with them and preferably do so in their own home. The benefits of the home visit are difficult to evaluate formally but experience suggests a number of important benefits:

1. Conditions at home can cause a number of problems notably hypothermia, fires, and falls.

2. The design and layout of the dwelling of a person who is suffering from a disabling disease have to be taken into account in assessment (see p. 160).

3. Housing problems can cause anxiety and depression (see p. 182).

4. A visit to the person's home helps to establish the relationship between doctor and patient. Cartwright and Anderson emphasized this:

> The number of home visits paid in the last year was clearly related to (the patient's) satisfaction with their care, to their views of their relationship with their doctor as being friendly rather than businesslike, to the assessment of whether or not they would consult their doctor about a personal problem and to whether they found their doctor an easy person to talk to?

However, home visits are time consuming and not only their effectiveness but their efficiency has to be assessed. This is something which each doctor has to decide for himself, in the context of all the other demands made on and possible uses of that scarcest of resources – time.

POVERTY AND POWERLESSNESS

Fundamental to the problems of elderly people is their poverty which reflects and perpetuates their powerlessness and low status. The basic retirement pension for those who have paid regular contributions into the National Insurance Fund over many years is one-tenth of the salary of the general practitioner or consultant. The social and political implications of their poverty are too complicated to discuss in this book in which we can simply attempt only to give some practical advice on how poverty can be mitigated (see p. 176). Nevertheless, poverty dominates the lives of many elderly people and the fact that older people are one of the deprived groups within our society influences their beliefs and attitudes and their health.

7 Prevention in old age

The scope for prevention in old age is considerable. The aging process cannot be prevented but the three other processes which cause problems in old age — disease, unfitness, and the social consequences of growing old — all offer opportunities for prevention. Each offers opportunities for primary, secondary, and tertiary prevention; that is complete prevention of the problem, early detection, and intervention, while the problem is at an early and treatable stage and effective intervention when problems are well established to prevent available complications (Table 7.1).

OPPORTUNITIES FOR PREVENTION

The consultation

The *aide-mémoire* suggested by Professor Harvard-Davis and Dr Nigel Stott as a means of using the full potential of the consultation is particularly useful with older patients among whom the need for advice on health promotion and the prevalence of continuing problems are greater and whose 'help-seeking behaviour' often needs modification, more commonly to encourage consultation than to encourage self-care, as is often the case with younger patients (Fig 7.1) (Stott and Davis 1979).

The appreciation of the 'exceptional potential of each primary care consultation' has been an important factor in the development of the case-finding approach to prevention, that is using any consultation initiated by a patient as an opportunity for the identification of risk factors and for health education – 'opportunistic health promotion'. There are ethical problems involved in this approach because the doctor is raising subjects which may not be a source of

A	B
Management of presenting problems	Modification of help-seeking behaviour
C	D
Management of continuing problems	Opportunistic health promotion

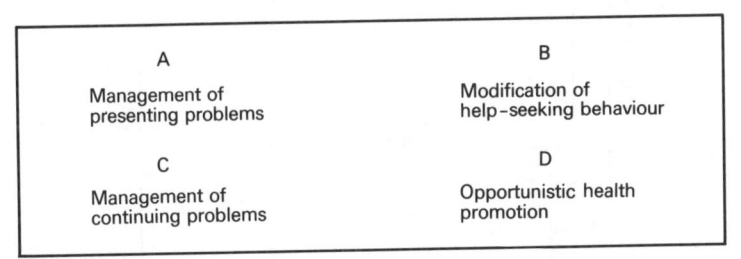

Fig. 7.1. The exceptional potential in each primary care consultation (Stott and Davis 1979).

Table 7.1. *The scope for prevention*

Problem	Example of primary prevention	Example of secondary prevention	Example of tertiary prevention
Disease	Prevention of obesity by dietary advice Prevention of stroke by treatment of high blood pressure	Early detection of heart block by 'case-finding' approach – i.e. – by enquiry about general health when patient consults for upper respiratory tract infection	Effective treatment of Parkinson's disease
Unfitness	Promotion of exercise in pre-retirement education Music and movement class in old people's homes	Advice on benefits of exercise given to person with arthritis during home visit to treat elderly spouse	Graduated exercise programme for patient with peripheral vascular disease
Social consequences of growing old	Generous pension policy Progressive housing policy Education of elderly people and relatives about benefits available	Discovery that old person is worried about housing and heating costs by enquiries made during course of consultation for review of medication prescribed for Parkinson's disease	Provision of improvement grants to instal inside toilet and prevent need for re-housing

concern to the patient and may create anxiety or suggest a fundamental change in the person's lifestyle. However, this type of activity is more acceptable when it develops in the course of a consultation initiated by a patient than when it has been initiated by the doctor, as occurs in formal screening programmes.

The importance of the contribution of the general practitioner as a health educator has been established in younger age groups but his impact is probably even greater with older patients because of the trust which older patients have in 'my doctor' and the effect which that trust has on compliance. The consultation is therefore a very effective medium for health education. Furthermore, it is also an efficient means of health promotion.

The case-finding approach has two major advantages over the screening approach – it avoids the need to arrange for the transport of elderly people to the screening clinic, if the clinic is used as the focus for screening, and it minimizes the amount of additional home visiting if it is decided to concentrate on home assessments.

The pre-retirement course

Another opportunity for prevention is offered by the retirement course, in which there is always a section on health. The Medical Advisory Panel of the Pre-Retirement Association have produced a useful guide for doctors invited to speak on such a course called *Third Age Health*. This can be obtained, with further reference and teaching material, from the Pre-Retirement Association, 19 Undine Street, London SW17 8PP.

Sometimes the organizers of pre-retirement courses find difficulty in recruiting doctors and enquiries from any doctor who is interested will be welcomed by the organizers of pre-retirement courses. They can be contacted locally through the Workers' Educational Association or by writing to the head office of the Pre-Retirement Association.

Old people's clubs

General practitioners and health visitors who work with well-defined populations in country areas and who are interested in educating older people about prevention health problems will find that old people's clubs present good opportunities for education. These clubs are moving away from the 'tea and bingo' type of activity and are becoming increasingly involved in education.

Professional and staff training

Much prevention can be done indirectly by the education of those who meet elderly people. Particularly important are the large number of people who receive very little training but who meet and have good relationships with large numbers of elderly people.

Ministers of religion.
Home helps.
Care assistants in old people's homes.

130 *Prevention in old age*

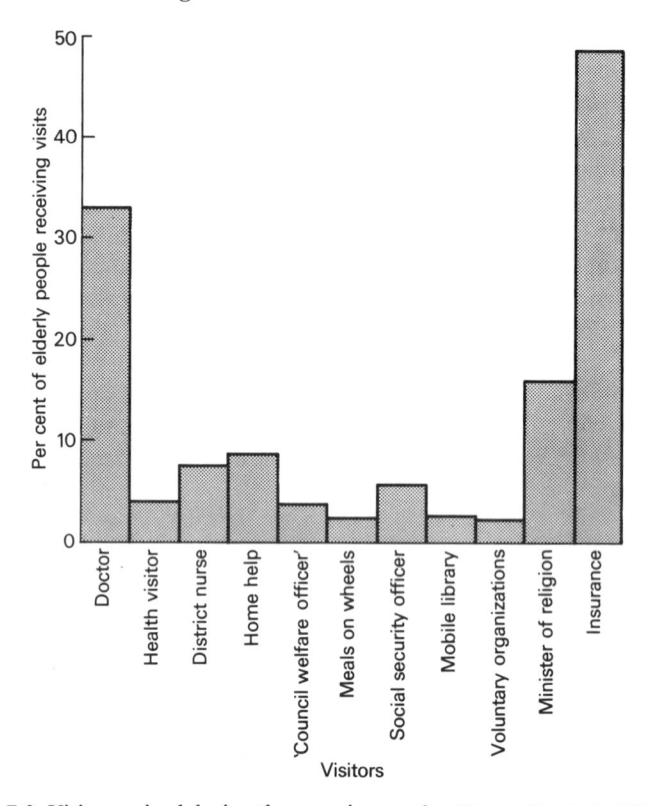

Fig. 7.2. Visits received during the past six months. (From Hunt, A. 1978).

Wardens of sheltered housing.
Volunteers who deliver meals on wheels and organize clubs and day centres.
Nursing auxiliaries.

The general practitioner, district nurse, and health visitor can make a very valuable contribution to the training of these workers by offering their help to those who organize the services. Anyone who visits an old person at home and who has a relationship with them should be considered as a possible health educator and supplied with the appropriate advice. The education of relatives is particularly important. It is interesting to note that the study *The Elderly At Home* found one other group who visit elderly people at home regularly, indeed the members of this group had visited a higher proportion of old people than general practitioners: perhaps we should try to establish closer links with the insurance men (Fig. 7.1).

IMPORTANT PRIMARY PREVENTIVE MESSAGES

Preventive measures will be discussed in many sections of this book; all the sections on disease and disability may be considered to be tertiary prevention. In this chapter we will focus on five important aspects of primary prevention, and in the next chapter secondary prevention will be discussed in more detail.

Keep active—use it or lose it

There is an increasing amount of good evidence that unfitness is a common cause of disability in old age and that elderly people can maintain fitness and become fitter by taking regular exercise. This applies not only to those who are free from disease – it applies even more to those old people who suffer from the common chronic diseases of old age.

Five aspects of fitness

There are five aspects of fitness, each of which begins with the letter S (Table 7.2). All the aspects of fitness can be improved, and all the complementary aspects of unfitness prevented or alleviated by exercise – no matter how old the person may be (Table 7.3).

In addition to encouraging people to maintain their level of fitness, and their relatives to allow them to do so, it is also important to encourage older people to try to become fitter by becoming more active. In this way they can become fitter and move nearer to their full potential (Fig. 7.3).

Again, it is particularly important to involve the spouse or relatives while planning the exercise programme to preclude a major cause of inactivity in old

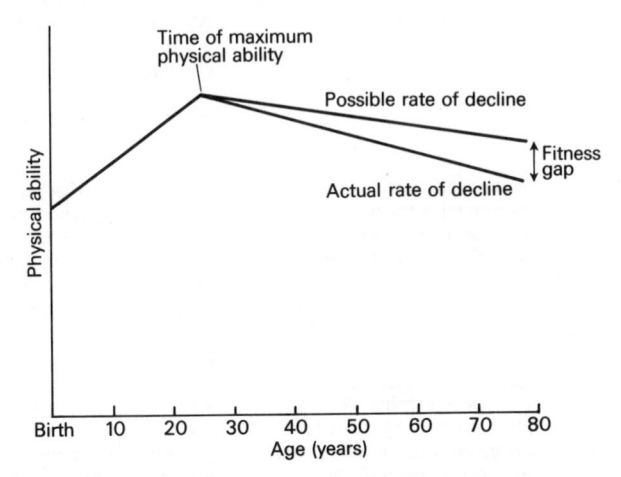

Fig. 7.3. The increasing gap between actual and possible levels of ability due to loss of fitness.

132 *Prevention in old age*

Table 7.2. *The five aspects of fitness*

Fitness	Unfitness
Strength	Weakness
Stamina	Breathlessness
Skill	Poor co-ordination
Suppleness	Stiffness
Self-esteem	Loss of self-confidence

Table 7.3. *Primary preventive benefits of exercise*

Aspect of fitness	Appropriate preventive measure for elderly people who can get about	Appropriate preventive measures for house-bound elderly people
Strength	Swimming, cycling, walking, and gardening. The important principle is that the old person should keep using her muscles for five or ten minutes after the first moment she feels that 'I'll just have a little rest now'	Housework and walking about the house, but the advice of a physio therapist is often necessary to give advice on those activities which the old person finds most difficult
Suppleness	Swimming is good but does not stretch all the muscles and joints. A keep-fit or music-and-movement, or Yoga class, is useful in giving the person the right type of exercise, and weekly stimulation, but very old person needs to be encouraged to stretch all the muscles and joints every day	The old person needs to be shown how to stretch all her muscles and joints gently and then encouraged to do the series of exercises every day
Stamina	The best advice is to 'get a little breathless every day in which ever way is most enjoyable'	The best approach is first to ask 'What make you breathless?' Almost every one knows, for some it is polishing a table, for others cleaning the floor, and the second step is to advise the housebound person that she should do something to become breathless every day
Skill	The more different types of exercise a person takes the better will be her co-ordination. Music-and-movement, keep-fit or Yoga are good for this but learning a new skill such as swimming or country dancing is also very helpful	The best form of occupational and physiotherapy is housework and the most important step is to ensure that other people do not try to 'help' the old person by doing things for her and removing the need for her to do housework herself
Self-esteem	Any type of exercise which is enthusiastically advocated and performed with enjoyment will have positive psychological benefits	Any type of exercise which is enthusiastically advocated and performed with enjoyment will have positive psychological benefits

Important primary preventive messages 133

age – namely the over-protective attitudes of other people. This is particularly important when the old person suffers from a chronic disease because of the widespread belief that exercise is harmful for such people.

Exercise and chronic disease

Exercise has been shown to be effective in the management of the diseases shown in Table 7.6.

When giving advice to patients and relatives about exercise it is important to be specific and give precise instructions about the duration, frequency, and, so far as is possible, intensity of exercise. In most cases it is possible to give advice clearly and safely without referral to a consultant or to a physiotherapist.

Exercise and acute illness

The effects of bed rest in young fit adults are striking. For example, one study showed a 28 per cent reduction in the cardiovascular fitness in five fit men (Saltin *et al.* 1968; Asher 1947) and this is a good indicator of the magnitude of the change which can occur in young people. Very elderly people who were not fit to start with not only lose fitness, particularly suppleness, even more quickly, but also find it harder to regain their fitness when the period of bed rest is over. It is therefore very important to minimize the amount of bed rest to as short a period as possible and precise instructions should be given to the patient and her relatives. If they are not specifically told about the need for early mobilization the period of bed rest will almost always be longer than is necessary, and the old person will receive an unnecessary setback. Advice is also needed during the period of 'convalescence' because the family may equate the term 'convalescence' with rest rather than with rehabilitation and take over tasks which the old person could perform before her illness, leading to a further loss of fitness. A complete review of an old person's recovery from an acute episode of illness should therefore include a comparison of her ability to perform household tasks before and after her illness and the objective should

Table 7.4. *Tertiary preventive effects of exercise*

Disease	Effect
Airways obstruction	Increased exercise tolerance
Peripheral arterial insufficiency	Increased walking distance
Obesity	Weight loss if exercise becomes a regular feature of daily life and is not accompanied by increased intake of food
Diabetes	'Insulin sparing' effect allows better control
Arthritis, stroke, and other muscular skeletal disorders	Less joint stiffness. Increased muscular strength. Reduction of pain

From Fentem and Bessey (1978).

Mental fitness

There is also evidence that some of the intellectual decline which is observed in old age is due not to the aging process but to a loss of fitness. Mental activity should therefore be encouraged, especially that which involves the old person's mind in interaction and conflict with other minds: argument is better than solitary study. As housework and self care are the best forms of physiotherapy and occupational therapy so normal conversation debate and argument is the best means of retaining and improving mental fitness. It is therefore important to try to prevent isolation (see p. 195) and to make sure that those people who meet the elderly person treat her as they treat their peers and do not underestimate her ability and thus ignore her right to be argued with and disagreed with (see p. 121).

'Be careful with home medicines'

The consumption of home medicines is very common in old age (Table 7.7).

Self care has much to commend it even in old age, but it can give rise to problems, notably delayed referral and side-effects. The side-effects of laxatives are especially common in older age groups. It is therefore necessary to emphasize a number of points about self medication when speaking to older people and their relatives:

1. Take care with any medicine, however harmless it may appear to be.
2. Always read carefully the direction folder provided with a medicine.
3. Never treat any symptom for longer than a week without consulting your doctor.
4. If a medicine which you have used according to instructions fails to have the desired effect, consult your doctor.
5. Keep medicines in a closed, dark cupboard in a cool place, out of the reach of children.
6. Do not keep medicines for longer than a year.
7. *Destroy completely* what is left of a medicine after you have finished with it. *Never throw medicines into the dustbin.*
8. If in doubt ask the advice of the pharmacist.

Table 7.5. *Self-medication in old age*

Percentage who had taken medication in two weeks before interview	Age group 65–74	Age group Over 75
Any medicine	82	92
Prescribed medicine	49	71
Home medicine	65	71

From Anderson, J. A. D. (1980). *Self-medication,* p. 24. MTP, Lancaster.

Alcohol abuse

This is probably becoming a more common problem, although some of the increase in observed prevalence is almost certainly due to increased awareness. The diagnosis, as at any age, can be very difficult if the patient tries to conceal their drinking but even when the old person does not try to conceal the amount she is consuming the cause of her problems may be missed because no-one thinks of it. Alcohol abuse must always be considered in the differential diagnosis:

Acute confusion
Chronic confusion
Memory failure
Behaviour problems
'Failing to cope'
Self-neglect
Anorexia

This list includes only a few of the ways in which alcohol abuse may present. The key diagnostic factor is usually that there has been an increase in the amount of alcohol consumed, although some old people develop problems without increasing their intake because their tolerance of alcohol declines owing to liver and brain failure.

When a drinking problem is suspected a number of questions arise:

What is the old person's opinion? Does she think she has a problem and is she willing to admit it?

What is the cause of the abuse? Is it isolation, or grief or depression?

Is the alcohol abuse causing any physical problems such as vitamin deficiency?

Should the aim be controlled drinking or complete abstinence?

if the analysis of the problem is difficult, referral to an Alcohol Treatment Unit is indicated, but most problems can be managed without referral. Few good studies on alcohol abuse in old age have been done, so it is difficult to give specific advice about the use of drugs or the objectives of treatment, but the most important step is to try to identify and then tackle the cause of the problem. It is always necessary to hold a case conference if it is decided to try to achieve either controlled drinking or abstinence so that every one who is involved is aware of the objectives. If this is not done the old person may be able to maintain her drinking by asking different people to buy quarter bottles of drink instead of relying on one person to buy a whole bottle.

'Take care of yourself'

Older people need advice on the steps they can take to maintain their body in good condition for two reasons. Firstly, because certain changes due to the aging process can cause problems which can be mitigated and secondly because some older people believe that there is little point in trying to look after their

136 *Prevention in old age*

body, believing that all the changes which take place are due to the aging process and that nothing can be done to prevent them.

Many diseases develop as the skin ages but even the healthy aging skin needs care and attention, particularly when the old person is unable to wash or dry herself thoroughly. Flexural intertrigo is very common in old age, for example under the breasts, and is accepted as normal by some old people. Elderly people should be taught about the need to dry their skin thoroughly each time they wash, if necessary by sitting with the skin exposed in a warm room rather than dressing immediately while still a little damp. The use of talcum powder should be encouraged. In addition the old person should be told that she should seek advice if her skin develops 'redness' or 'soreness' or 'itchiness'.

Advice on hair care is also helpful as disorders of the scalp can cause distress. Regular hairwashing is the best maintenance measure, preferably by a visit to the hairdresser if the person cannot manage it herself, because of the social benefits of the trip. The District Nurse, or more commonly the Nursing Auxiliary, is able to help housebound people, but even if the Nurse does become involved an attempt should be made to restore the old person's mobility and self-esteem to the point at which a visit to the hairdresser's can be achieved (Fig. 7.3).

Eyes

Every old person should be advised to go to see an optician every two years, even if she does not notice any change in her vision. Many old people accept correctable refractive problems because they assume 'it's just old age'. If problems develop before two years have elapsed it is obviously important for the old person to see the optician sooner. It is usually fairly easy to arrange voluntary transport to the opticians for the test and, if necessary, the fitting, because it is a limited but rewarding task for a volunteer to do.

Elderly people who receive supplementary pension can get National Health Service glasses free. The optician holds a stock of 'Form F1' which should be completed by the supplementary pensioner (see p. 81).

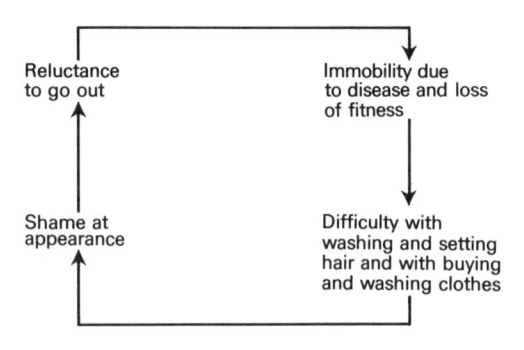

Fig. 7.4.

Ears (see p. 35)

There is little that the elderly people can do to preserve their ability to hear but they should be encouraged to seek help as soon as they notice a deterioration in their hearing, for example inability to hear the telephone ringing or to hear normal conversation when there is some background noise. The benefits of early referral are twofold:

1. Accurate assessment and, if possible, treatment, with ear-syringing the most common means of effective treatment.

2. Education about the way to cope with a loss of hearing and, even more difficult, with the unhelpful approach of other people.

Teeth and dentures

Those who still have teeth should be encouraged to try to keep them with the advice being the same as for younger people.

'Remember that sugar causes decay. If you like sweets limit your consumption to a chocolate or two after meals and then brush your teeth.'

'Brush your teeth thoroughly at least once a day.'

'Try to see a dentist regularly even if you have no symptoms. If toothache or painful or bleeding gums develop try to see a dentist as soon as you can.'

People who have dentures also need advice. In addition to advice on the cleaning of dentures they need to be told:

'Gums shrink quickly when the first set of dentures is being worn. Go back and see your dentist six months after you have had your false teeth fitted.'

'Try to see a dentist once every two years even though your dentures are comfortable.'

'If your dentures feel uncomfortable or loose or painful try to see a dentist as soon as possible.'

Unfortunately many elderly people have great difficulty in putting such advice into action because of the difficulty in finding a dentist willing to treat elderly people 'on the NHS'. If an informed approach to one's own dentist or to friends who are dentists is unsuccessful, the District Dental Officer may be able to suggest a dentist who would be willing to see the old person. Home visits are much less useful than an examination in the surgery but voluntary transport is usually possible to arrange. Elderly people who receive a supplementary pension or who have a low income can get free treatment and dentures. The dentist keeps 'Form F1D' which the old person should complete. It is essential to emphasize to old people and to their relatives that the dentist appreciates that the treatment he is going to give is not private treatment before the course of treatment starts.

8 Family problems

> I find the services are very helpful in my part of the country. After I had had my breakdown they all helped me wonderfully with mother.

THE MODERN FAMILY

It is widely believed that the modern family 'doesn't care as much' for its elders as it did in the past. This belief is not new and the view that the family does not care for its elderly members has been expressed for many years.

> The Report of the Poor Law Commissioners of 1832 stated categorically that 'the duty of supporting parents and children in old age or infirmity is so strongly enforced by our natural feelings that it is well performed even among savages, and almost always so in a nation deserving the name of civilised. We believe that England is the only European country in which it is neglected'.
>
> The next great Royal Commission on the Poor Laws and the Relief of Distress, which sat between 1905 and 1909, also emphasized 'the disinclination of relatives to assist one another'.

There is, however, no evidence that families care less well for their elders than they did. It is probably true that a higher proportion of elderly people were respected and venerated in the past. The reason for the respect and veneration was, however, not so much their age as the fact that there was no compulsory retirement and elderly parents continued to manage the family business until they died. The children who were thus held in economic dependency until their thirties or forties had to respect the parents on whom they were economically dependent more than modern children who are less dependent but they were not necessarily more caring or loving. Indeed the opposite was often true as economic dependence frequently produces resentment and sometimes hatred, as still happens in some farming communities in Britain in which the son is not allowed to sign cheques on his own, and has to consult his father on all business matters, until the father dies.

Many elderly parents were aware of such feelings of their children and were afraid to relinquish their power – the fate of King Lear was not uncommon.

Rich old people were often respected and powerful but the fate of poor and impotent old people offers a more accurate indication of society's attitudes. Data are scarce for the nineteenth century, but it is possible to calculate the proportion of old people living in institutions throughout this century and these

Table 8.1. *Proportion of elderly people permanently institutionalized*

Year	Percentage of people aged 65 in institutions
1911	5.17
1921	3.39
1931	2.91
1952	2.10
1961	2.79
1973	2.88

From Moroney (1976, p. 48).
The proportion of people aged over 65 who are very elderly has increased since 1911 and this increase accounts for the slight increase in the total number of people institutionalized between 1952 and 1973.

data show that the proportion of old people who were permanently institutionalized in 1911 was almost twice that in 1971 (Table 8.1).

Peter Laslett, one of the historians who has done much to dispel the belief that there was ever a 'Golden Age' for old people, wrote that it is 'unjustifiable to assume that the aged were always cherished by their families and by their kinfolk in the pre-industrial era'. The modern family cares as well as the family in any previous era (Moroney 1976).

Reluctant relatives

Every doctor is, of course, able to cite cases in which the family has refused to care for an elderly person, and it may be that the number of such cases is increasing as the number of old people increase. There are three common reasons why families refuse to help an elderly relative.

Firstly, they may refuse to become involved because they fear that the acceptance of any responsibility will be the thin end of the wedge and that they will eventually be asked to assume full responsibility. This fear can be overcome if the relatives are assured that they have no legal responsibility to take the old person to live with them, that no-one expects them to do this, and that they should not feel guilty if they do not want to do so.

Secondly, relatives may refuse to help because they feel no moral obligation to do so. If children do not feel motivated to help it may be because of the character of the old person. Not all old people are nice old people: many are self-centred and wish to dominate others. Such changes are not the natural consequences of aging and people who have these characteristics in old age were often similar when they were younger. They were self-centered and dominating to young people and showed their children little love when they were young. The children of such people may feel little obligation towards their elderly parents and their indifference or hostility is understandable. The child's reluctance to help may be aggravated by guilt about her indifference or hostility and the general practitioner's assurance that such feelings are natural may reduce her guilt and allow her to help her parent more easily.

Thirdly, some families refuse to continue caring not because they do not care for the elder but because they are exhausted. They were originally loving but have not had a holiday, or even an evening out together, for years and have coped with incontinent laundry without support. Such families do not give up because of the existence of the Welfare State: they give up because they have been offered too little help too late (Isaacs 1971).

Practical difficulties in visiting and helping

Finally, it should be remembered that there are many practical problems why relatives do not visit more often than they do. In the survey of the Elderly at Home (Hunt 1978) 26.8 per cent of old people said that they would like relatives to visit more often; the reasons why they did not are given in Table 8.2.

Table 8.2. *Reasons why relatives do not visit more often*

Reasons	Percentage
Lives abroad	16.4
Lives too far away in Great Britain	47.9
Family commitments	19.0
Work commitments	17.7
Health problems due to old age of relatives	24.6
Too busy	4.8
Doesn't want to come	4.5
Expense	23.3
Other reasons	6.0
No reason given	7.4

From Hunt, A. (1978). *The elderly at home,* HMSO, London.

The modern family is therefore often unable to help although it is willing. Relatives who try to help often have problems and need help themselves.

CAUSE OF RELATIVES' PROBLEMS

The old person's disability

The problems commonly experienced by relatives were clearly revealed by a study of fifty families conducted in London in 1974 (Table 8.3).

When relatives seek help attention is usually focused on the old person. It is she who is presented as 'the problem' and it is by modification of her condition or her circumstances that the relatives envisage an amelioration of their own condition. It is usually the relatives who make the first contact, often without the knowledge of the old person, describing their difficulties with reference to the old person's disabilities or behaviour. Their complaint may be vague initially, for example they may say that they 'Can't cope any longer' or that they 'can't go on'. They may be much more specific, for example complaining about incontinence, continued mumbling, or physical dependence, and careful questioning almost always pinpoints certain specific areas which are the major

Table 8.3. *Behavioural and self-care problems*

	Frequency (% of cases)	Tolerance (% of supporters able to tolerate problems)
Sleep disturbance	62	16
Night wandering	24	24
Micturition	24	17
Shouting	10	20
Incontinence of faeces	56	43
Incontinence of urine	54	81
Falls	58	52
Inability to get out of bed unaided	52	35
Inability to get into bed unaided	50	40
Inability to get on commode unaided	36	22
Inability to get off commode unaided	38	21
Dangerous, irresponsible behaviour	32	38
Inability to walk unaided	18	33
Inability to walk at all	16	13
Personality conflicts	26	54
Physically aggressive behaviour	18	44
Inability to dress unaided	44	77
Inability to wash and/or shave unaided	54	93
Inability to communicate	16	50
Daytime wandering	12	33
Inability to manage stairs unaided	10	60
Inability to feed unaided	12	67
Blindness	2	0
Restriction of social life	42	57
Inability to leave dependant for more than one hour	28	71
Stairs within accommodation	26	85
Financial disadvantage	4	0
Other	4	0

Sanford, J. R. A. (1975): Tolerance of debility in elderly dependants by relatives at home. *Br. Med. J.* **ii**, 471–3.

problems even though the initial complaint is that 'everything' is wrong. It is, however, very important to view the problem as a family problem rather than as simply a geriatric problem arising solely from the old person's physical or mental condition. Careful assessment of the whole family is as important as careful assessment of the old person.

Relatives seek professional help when they can no longer cope without it. The timing of the referral is determined not only by the severity of the old person's problems but it is also a function of the family's ability to cope. In some instances the reason for the referral is solely due to a change in the old person's condition; when, for example, the old person suffers a severe stroke. In other cases the reason for the referral is solely due to a change in the condition of one or more of the supporters; when, for example, the active member of an elderly married couple has a heart attack and the disabled partner has to be admitted to hospital even though there has been no change in her condition. In most cases, however, both factors are present: the old person's disability has been steadily increasing and the family's ability to cope

142 *Family problems*

has been steadily decreasing until the point is reached at which they can no longer cope without help.

Problems of the principal carer

Within each family there is always one member who is more closely involved than the others. It is more often a daughter than a son, and more often a 'blood' relation than an in-law although many daughters-in-law do more than their husbands. The person principally involved may be termed the carer with the other members of the family being termed the supporters and the old person may be referred as a result of some change in the condition of the carer or the supporters or because of some social pressure outside the family.

The carer's ability to cope may be affected by his own state of health, or by his relationship with the elder, or by his relationship with the supporters or by outside pressures or by a combination of these factors. The sons and daughters of elderly people with multiple problems are often middle-aged and sometimes elderly. Commonly they are in their forties and fifties but many are in their sixties and some are even older. Physical disease of a type which impairs their ability to care for their elderly parent is therefore not uncommon. Arthritis and backache are particularly difficult if the parent requires lifting. Other chronic diseases which do not directly affect the tasks which the carer is required to perform may also be relevant if they tire the supporter. Thus someone with severe diabetes may reach a point at which the demands and needs of her elderly relative become intolerable even though the diabetes does not directly impair the carer's ability to perform such tasks as are required. Mental illness, which may of course be caused by the burden of caring, also reduces the carer's ability to cope and it is important to identify the carer and to ensure that she is as fit as she can be.

The nature of the relationship between carer and elder is also relevant. If the two are parent and child the latter may have considerable difficulty. When a child becomes an adult in a social sense by achieving economic independence and the age of twenty-one her relationship with her parents changes and they usually relate to one another as unrelated adults relate to one another, for example discussing political issues or social issues, such as homosexuality, without any more embarrassment or difficulty than they would have with strangers they met on a train. However, aspects of the parent–child relationship remain, for example the expectation of the parent that he will be obeyed and the deference of the child to parental opinion, and in some such relationships the dominance of the parent and the defence of the child remain marked even though the child is in her forties or fifties. In general, the degree of parental dominance in old age reflects the degree of dominance which the parent had over the child when younger, and although it may increase it may also decrease until the child dominates the parent. Even if the parent is not overtly domineering the child may find it difficult to correct her parent when he makes a mistake or behaves in a way which is upsetting, for example when he speaks

Table 8.4.

Methods used by adult children to control their elderly parents (American study)	Percentage
Screamed and yelled	40
Used physical restraint	6
Forced feeding or medication	6
Threatened to send to nursing home	6
Threatened with physical force	4
Hit or slapped	3

From Steinmetz, S. K. (1981). *Elder Abuse: Aging,* Jan.–Feb., 6–10.

of his deceased wife or when he breaks wind loudly when there are guests present. Similarly, the strength of the emotional bond, of the love, between child and parent does not change naturally with age although the child may grow increasingly angry and resentful if she feels that she is being exploited by her elderly parent or feels trapped by her parent's dependence on her. The tension may be expressed in various ways as one study in America revealed (Table 8.4). The elderly people had their own means of retaliation and resistance (Table 8.5).

Table 8.5.

Methods used by elderly people to control their adult children	Percentage
Scream and yell	43
Pout or withdraw	47
Refuse food or medication	16
Manipulate, cry, and use physical or mental disability	32
Hit, slap, throw objects	22
Call police or others for imagined threats	10

From Steinmetz, S. K. (1981). *Elder Abuse: Aging,* Jan.–Feb., 6–10.

Problems of other members of the family

A carer's ability to cope may be affected by members of the family other than the old person, notably the carer's spouse and children.

Husbands

Because it is more common for daughters to be carers the spouse involved is more often a husband although the difficulties discussed in this section are equally apposite to cases in which the old person lives with, or near, her married son who provides most of the care.

If the relationship between the old person and the son-in-law has always been unsatisfactory it is likely to deteriorate if the old person comes to live with the family. However, even relationships which were initially good may become soured as the old person requires increasing amounts of care from his or her daughter. The husband may become jealous of, and angry with, the old person and may also become angry with his wife for giving her parent priority. He may feel guilty about these feelings, as the wife may feel guilty about neglecting her husband. Furthermore, because the old person is often present, husband and wife may not have the opportunity to discuss these feelings and they may therefore become more intense.

Problems between husband and wife which are unrelated to the old person, for example sexual problems, may also have an affect on the daughter's ability to cope. So may her concern about her husband's financial problems or difficulties at work and all these factors have to be considered when assessing a family which has referred an old person because they can no longer cope with her.

Children

The relationship between children and grandparents is often easier than the relationship of either with the middle generation but even when there is an easy relationship between grandparents and grandchildren family difficulties may occur. The old person may 'spoil' the children, that is, allow them to behave in a manner which has been expressly forbidden by parents: even worse, while indulging the children in one way, the old person may be criticising some other aspect of their upbringing – 'I think it's wrong to let children stay out as late as that'.

The relationship between old and young is not always good, particularly in adolescence during which the young person's need for space and solitude may be restricted by the presence of a grandparent who complains about noise, dress, manners, attitudes, and values, and is shocked and offended when the young person answers back in a way which 'would never have happened in my day', and this may be taken by the middle generation as a criticism of them, as indeed it often is.

Problems of single sons and daughters

The problems of single daughters and single sons merit special mention. The carer who is a member of a family may have problems of the types described in the previous sections but a family is a source of support not only to the old person but to the carer. Single daughters and single sons do not have this type of support, they have no-one to reassure and to comfort them when the old person has been difficult. Neither do they have people in the household who can introduce other topics of conversation or divert their attention from the problem of caring. Social isolation and loneliness are particularly common but all the practical problems which families have with elderly people, problems such as incontinence or exhaustion, are a greater burden for the single carer. In addition her problems – there are more single daughters then sons in this role – with respect to housing and finance are much greater for the old person may be the owner or tenant of the dwelling they share and if the single daughter does not work the sole income of the household will be Social Security.

It is very helpful to try to ascertain how the single daughter came to be the carer. In some cases she will never have left home, and in others she will have returned home when the old person became disabled. Some of those who return do so very willingly but others return only as a result of sustained pressure by other, married siblings, and regrettably by professionals including doctors. Single daughters may be subjected to, and succumb to, moral blackmail – 'your mother's not really safe to be left alone now, you know' – and return home harbouring resentment to others which may impair her relationship with her parent.

Living arrangements

The distance which now separates many old people and their relatives creates problems for both. It limits the help which the relatives can give and increases their anxiety. The ideal arrangement for most households would be for the generations to live close to one another. Unfortunately, because this is difficult to arrange, the old person may move in with her son or daughter and this can lead to an increase in tension and create new problems.

PREVENTION OF FAMILY PROBLEMS

Primary prevention

An effective means of primary prevention of a common cause of problems is to help the family and the old person to decide that it would be better to live near one another than to live in the same household and then to help them implement that decision. However, it is rarely possible to do this for two reasons. Firstly, the general practitioner is rarely involved in this type of decision until it has been made and implemented. The first he knows about the decision is often the family's request that he take their elderly relative on to his list. The second reason is that even if the general practitioner is involved and advises the family that it will be easier if the old person lives near them rather than with them, it is usually impossible to arrange this unless the old person has enough money to buy her own dwelling. Most local authorities give low priority to housing applications from elderly people from another part of the country, even when they wish to return to the place where they were born. Some refuse even to accept applications from any old people who live outside their area. The family should ask the housing department for the names and addresses of any housing associations which have, or are building, properties in the district because the latter usually have less restrictive rules than local authorities and are more willing to try to help elderly people move to live near their relatives. Even if it does not prove possible to arrange for the old person to move to live near members of her family it should not be regarded as being inevitable that the old person should therefore move to live with them. It may be possible and preferable to help the old person to live on in her own home by improving her health and providing more services. Sometimes the general practitioner has to take an active part in discouraging an old person from moving if he feels that undue pressure is being exerted on her by worried relatives or that one member of the family, usually a single daughter, is being blackmailed by her siblings and their spouses to move in with the old person or to have her to live in her house.

If it is decided that the old person is to come to live with her family the best policy is to advise the two parties to try living together for three to six months, but again this is a policy of perfection which is not always possible to follow, for the old person may have to relinquish her council tenancy, thus burning her boats, if she wishes to move in with her daughter or son for a few months. Once the decision has definitely been made it is important to help the family reach an agreement about living arrangements.

Although the members of most families would have great difficulty in analysing and describing the contracts which exist in the family, the rituals which individuals and the whole family observe, and the territory which each member of the family occupies are features of family life, which evolve slowly and imperceptibly. A new member of a family disrupts the contracts, she interrupts rituals, invades the territories of the family which she joins, but the amount of disturbance can be minimized if the family sets out rules or guidelines governing the relationship between the old person and the other members of the family. It is useful to discuss and decide on arrangements about:

1. Territory: no matter how well the two parties think they 'get on' as a result of visits which the old person has made, permanent residence is much more difficult, but by arranging a period of time each day when the old person and other members of the family keep apart, by the old person staying in her room for example, problems can be prevented.

2. Meals: mealtimes are a source of conflict and without banishing the elder from the meal table it is possible to suggest that the nuclear family have at least one meal alone every day.

3. Social life: both the old person and the nuclear family need time and privacy to see their own friends.

4. Holidays: in some families the old person and the nuclear family holiday happily together but holidays may provide the caring family not only with a useful break from work but also with a useful break from the old person.

5. Finance: the contribution which the old person should make to household expenses should be clearly set out and agreed.

6. Help with housework: the old person may easily assume certain jobs but it can be helpful to decide on which jobs should be done by which member of the household. The old proverb about 'Two women in the one kitchen' is wise and the prevention of tension in the kitchen can prevent tension in the family.

The earlier this is done the easier it will be. It is much less upsetting to suggest to an old person that she spend every Sunday evening in her own room before she moves in, than to make the same suggestion after she has been living in the house for six months. Families may need some encouragement to take this approach because they may feel that it would indicate that they did not love one another if they were to discuss a set of rules as though they were drawing up a business contract. They may be helped to do so if it is emphasized that there are rules and contracts in every family but these are often unspoken because they have evolved over the course of many years and the only reason that it is necessary to speak about them is when a new family order is suddenly created by an old person joining it. When family problems are developing this approach can also be helpful and it is a technique which can be used in secondary prevention.

In addition, relatives need information and education about the problems of looking after elderly relatives and the services which are available to help them. Unfortunately those who are most in need are often least able to benefit from this approach which makes it even more important that all those who meet elderly people and their relatives are alert to the problems which can arise and the way in which they can be prevented or relieved so that they can practise secondary prevention.

Secondary prevention

A programme of surveillance of certain vulnerable old people which is initiated by the general practitioner is an effective means of prevention (see p. 205). The criteria of vulnerability of old people who live alone have been discussed and these relate very much to disability but a family with an old person living with them should also be considered a vulnerable unit and included in a surveillance programme. It is possible to do much of this by using consultations with the old person or other members of the family appropriately. Even though the reason for consultation has, or appears to have, no connection with the fact that the patient is a member of an extended family it provides a useful opportunity for discussing problems and difficulties. It is possible to raise this subject with a daughter easily by saying that it is normal for the arrival of an old person to cause some difficulties and it is normal for the old person and the younger members of the household to find difficulty in being frank with one another. Similarly, the old person can be assured that difficulties and communication are commonly difficult. If the old person is included in a surveillance because she is receiving regular prescriptions the consultation arranged for review of medication offers a good opportunity for this type of discussion but all the members of the family need to be given the opportunity to talk and sometimes husband and wife need the opportunity to talk on their own. The *aide mémoire* suggested by Dr Stott and Professor Davis is a useful means of practising anticipatory care and can be used when either the old person or her relatives consult (see p. 133).

If this case-finding approach is practised by general practitioner, district nurse, and health visitor and encouraged among those who meet elderly people, for example social workers, problems can often be anticipated and dealt with before they become severe.

Tertiary prevention

Finally, it is important to emphasize that tertiary prevention is almost always possible. Even when the family implacably or angrily demands permanent institutionalization as 'the only answer' it is usually possible to prevent rejection of the old person and a breakdown of the family by reducing the elder's disability and arranging for regular relief. The general practitioner's task may be made easier if the family is told firmly that permanent institutionalization is not a feasible proposition by a consultant in geriatric medicine or a consultant psychiatrist. Increasingly, however, general practitioners have to support families looking after old people who should, in the opinion of the relatives, the general practitioner and the hospital consultant, live in an institution. In some cases it is clear which institution should accept the old person, in others the old person, her relatives and general practitioner are pushed from pillar to post being told by the hospital that she is 'too fit' to be admitted and being told by Social Services that she is 'too frail'. In such cases the objective of the doctor is to prevent the carer and the old person from suffering too much.

ASSESSMENT OF FAMILY PROBLEMS

Assessment checklist
(a) Assessment of the old person:
   1. Physical condition.
   2. Mental state.
   3. Attitude towards 'the problem'.
(b) Assessment of the principal carer:
   1. Physical and mental health.
   2. Relationship with the old person.
   3. Relationships with other members of the family.
   4. Social problems.
(c) Assessment of the other relatives:
   1. Physical and mental health.
   2. Relationship with the old person.
   3. Relationship with the carer.
   4. Social problems.

In all aspects of assessment changes in time are particularly important. It is, for example, very helpful to assess not only the current state of the relationship between the elder and carer but also to try to determine the nature of the relationship during the preceding thirty years. A careful analysis of the timing of the referral is usually illuminating—why was the problem not referred a week ago or a month ago? The timing may be simply explained by a deterioration in the old person's condition but if that has not changed significantly in the last week or month it is probable that some factor other than the old person's condition is more important. A more detailed consideration of the days or even the hours before referral is often useful if one focuses not on the problem referred but on the manner in which the decision to refer was made. With whom did the person who actually referred the problem discuss whether or not she should refer the problem?

What do they expect to happen as a result of referral? It is important to try to ascertain the expectations of the family as soon as possible and to disillusion the relatives as soon as possible if their expectations are impossible to meet or inappropriate.

It may be difficult for members of the family to accept that a social or personal problem which has nothing to do with the old person has affected their tolerance of her. They may not reveal such problems because they do not see what link they could have with the problem they are having with the old person and therefore do not see why they should reveal them to a doctor they have called in to arrange for the institutionalization of their elder. If they do recognize that problems at work or marital problems could be affecting their attitude towards the old person they may be reluctant to admit it, thinking that they might be criticised for allowing their problems to have an effect on the old person. It may therefore be easier for the family to answer a question in which they are asked if the worry and strain of caring for the old person is affecting their ability to cope with difficulties in the family or at work than to answer a question which asks if there is any social or personal problem which could be reducing their ability to cope with the old person's difficulties. The latter approach gives the impression that the doctor supports the family's contention that the sole problem is the old person but even if the general practitioner suspects that it is not the case this approach may be a more effective means of eliciting information than suggesting that the referral results from the family's failings.

Reaching agreement

Having decided on the most important problem or problems it is necessary to persuade both the old person and the family to agree that the general practitioner's formulation identifies the main problems and the most practicable solutions. The doctor may decide that the problem which the relatives referred—the old person's physical or mental state—is the only significant problem and have to convince an old person who maintains that he is 'all right' that things cannot continue as they are. In other cases the doctor may decide that the problem identified by the family is of no more than minor importance compared with a marital problem or some other social difficulty which is unrelated to the old person. In such cases he has to dissuade the relatives from their beliefs that the old person is 'the problem' and that institutionalization of the elder is the only solution to their difficulties. In most cases, however, both the old person and the relatives have to accept some modification of the view which they held at the time of referral: the old person has to agree that everything is not 'all right', and the relatives have to agree that the problem does not only result from the old person's disability. Similarly both the old person and the family usually have to agree to accept some modification of their views as to the solution of the problems.

Negotiations with families involve a good deal of diplomacy. The doctor must take care that he is not seen as being on one side or the other. When intervening in a family in which tensions are running high there is a risk that he may be considered to be another conspirator by the old person while the relatives see him as being on the side of the old person because he does not appear to appreciate their burden fully. The doctor acts like a conciliator and arbitrator in an industrial dispute. He has to aim to reach a compromise which both parties will agree is acceptable although it fully satisfies the expectations of neither party. It is essential for both parties to feel that their problems and position have been understood and that the compromise suggestion is fair to both parties. They should also feel that they are being fairly treated by the health and social services. If they cannot be given all the help they think they should receive because resources are short this should be made clear to them. Most families respond responsibly if told that it is only by offering a little help to each family that the many families in difficulty can be helped. At the end of the interview the family may still feel that they are being unfairly treated by society in having to carry such a heavy burden but feel that they are being fairly treated by the general practitioner and the hospital or social services.

If they do feel this they can be advised to write to a member of the health authority or their councillor, or to the Member of Parliament if these routes fail. It is essential to help the family distinguish between the unfairness of their treatment by society and the fairness of their treatment by the general practitioner because their trust in him is necessary if he is going to try to change attitudes.

COPING WITH COMMON PROBLEMS

The first and most valuable step is often to let the relatives talk about their problems and feelings. The opportunity to express hostile feelings and to be reassured that they are understandable is often of considerable benefit. However, it is always appropriate to see if the burden of the relatives can be relieved.

Physical exhaustion
Sometimes the person caring for a disabled elder develops some disease herself and it should not be automatically assumed that exhaustion results from the

burden of caring. Her state of health should therefore be reviewed before attempting to relieve her of some of the burden (Grad and Sansbury 1965).

If nothing can be done to strengthen the carer by improving her health an attempt should be made to spare her from some of the more tiring tasks. Home help is usually associated with old people who live alone but it can be a very effective use of home help to relieve the person who is caring from some of the washing, or housework, and home help organizers are willing to accept such requests. District nurses can also be very effective in the prevention and relief of exhaustion if used to spare a supporter from the burden, and in some cases the embarrassment, of bathing or dressing the old person.

Great relief can also be offered by regular day care, either in an old people's home or in hospital but a common difficulty is reluctance on the part of the old person. Sometimes the old person does not realize how much the carer is suffering and the doctor may have to tell her or, preferably, help the carer to tell her and help her to appreciate that although she feels 'all right' her refusal to go to day hospital or day care is affecting other people. This can be difficult for both parties. The carer, for example a single daughter, may fear that her mother will take this to mean that she no longer loves her, or fear that her mother will say that she feels rejected just to make the daughter feel guilty, and the mother may feel guilty or rejected. If it proves difficult to help such issues to be discussed it may be useful to involve a social worker (see p. 102).

Day care does not, however, give relief at night and the admission of the old person to an institution can help relieve the carer's exhaustion more effectively. The admission of the old person to allow her supporters to go on their annual holiday is a good use of resources but many families need help more often, for example three days every fortnight or for two weeks every three months. If the old person is adversely affected by such a programme, or by regular attendance at day hospital or day centre, these effects have to be balanced against the benefits which the family, and indirectly the elder, are receiving. It may be necessary to stop a programme of regular relief because the relocation effect is too great but it is usually possible to overcome or reduce the problems of relocation (see p. 109). As with attendance at day hospital there may be difficulty in persuading the old person to accept the need for admission and this may require the doctor or a social worker to spend some time with the elderly person and her supporters.

Whatever the pattern of relief offered it is essential that it be regular and assured. The family needs to feel that they have absolute security in the arrangement, to be confident that for three days every fortnight, or whatever, the elder will be admitted for as long as the family feel the need for relief, for as long as the elder lives if necessary. The general practitioner should try to ensure that the hospital or old people's home makes a commitment to regular relief and that the family appreciate this, because it can greatly reduce the tension within the family which contributes to exhaustion and breakdown.

One factor contributes to exhaustion so commonly that it merits special mention – sleep disturbance.

Sleep disturbance

Many elderly people sleep less well than they did when younger. This is not a consequence of aging but of certain changes in life-style, for example a decrease in day-time activity and an increase in the time spent sleeping during the day, with the result that the person wakes more often during the night. The fact that physically dependent elderly people may be put to bed at an early hour because they must retire when staff are available to help them may also result in night waking and physical disease may disturb sleep, for example the elderly person may be woken by painful joints or by the need to micturate.

The change in sleep pattern worries some elderly people and their anxiety may worry their relatives but the elder's sleeplessness can have more direct effects on the well being of relatives who live with her. The knowledge that the old person gets up during the night gives rise to anxiety if she is unsteady and has a history of falls, or if it is thought that she will try to cook something or light the fire. Even though the old person never wakes and never rises the relatives' anxiety that she may do so can seriously disturb their own sleep and contribute to her exhaustion. The relative may sleep more easily and therefore be less tired if she can be sure that she will wake as soon as the old person rises.

In other families the principal problem is not the relatives' anxiety but the noise created by the old person when she gets up and flushes the toilet or goes downstairs and opens and closes cupboard doors looking for something to eat. This type of behaviour may be tolerable if it is only once a night but it can become intolerably tiring if it is three or four times a night.

To reduce the problem the first step is to try to increase the duration of the elder's sleep and to try to reduce night waking. Hypnotics are sometimes useful (p. 93), but before prescribing a hypnotic the following measures should be tried:

1. Encourage physical and mental activity: advising walks, swimming, and cycling for active elders who are independent and day care for those who are more dependent.

2. Discourage 'naps' and 'dozing off' during the day.

3. Advise the old person to retire to bed later, but remember that the reason for an early bedtime may be to give the relatives time to themselves.

4. Encourage the old person and her relatives to develop a regular pattern of behaviour before going to bed; for example, a warm milk drink, such as Horlicks, Ovaltine, or Bournvita at 9.30, followed by a peaceful half-hour at the fire, reading a magazine or book, with a very small sherry or rum at 10.15 before retiring to a warm bed in a warm room. This type of behaviour can be very conducive to sleep, providing it is performed every night so that it becomes a pre-sleep ritual.

It is also important to try to minimize the disturbance caused by the need to micturate. Some old people will always wake to pass water at night but severe restriction of fluids should be discouraged. It is more important to try to provide the means by which they can pass water quietly, easily, and safely in their own room, providing a light which can be easily reached and a urinal or commode. If the old person is in the habit of making a cup of tea a flask and a tin of biscuits beside the light may preclude the need to go downstairs.

Interference with social life

Many of the people who have elderly people living with them have to limit their social life. Going out in the evening may become a problem and the general practitioner should enquire about this. In some cases there may be no need for the carer to be afraid of leaving the old person alone and all that may be required is to help her reduce to tolerable levels the anxieties which she feels about leaving the old person. She may be anxious about falls or setting fire to the house; she may be anxious about what neighbours will say; or she may be anxious that the old person will make life more difficult by complaining or implying that she feels neglected if she is left, a type of emotional tie which is particularly difficult for single sons and daughters (see p. 155). If it is impossible for the elderly person to be left alone, either because she is at great risk or because the carer cannot be induced to leave her, attempts should be made to arrange for someone to sit in. The local branch of the British Red Cross Society or the St. John Ambulance Association may be able to provide a volunteer or the local office of Age Concern may know of a suitable volunteer, preferably someone who can do the task regularly enough to get to know, and be known by, the old person. If such a scheme does not exist a general practitioner can, in conjunction with these voluntary organizations, take the initiative in setting one up (see p. 168).

Some families also have difficulty in entertaining because of the presence of an elderly relative whom it is feared will embarrass their guests. In some cases this is true and one of the benefits of an admission of short duration is that it allows the family to entertain freely. This is not the only means by which a family's social life can be improved however. All that may be necessary is for the old person to be told that her relatives need time to themselves and that they need time to see their own friends alone. Often relatives find it impossible to say this themselves and it may be necessary for the general practitioner, district nurse, or health visitor to say it or, better, to help the relatives to say it in a manner in which the old person appreciates the validity of their point and does not feel rejected or insulted.

The difficulty which close relatives have in being open with one another contributes to another of the major problems – behaviour problems.

Behaviour problems

It is easy to appreciate how some types of behaviour prove intolerable to relatives. The old person who urinates in the corner of the room or walks about naked is obviously difficult for the family to cope with, but it is often patterns of behaviour which one would think could be tolerated which are described as being intolerable. The noise the old person makes with his false teeth, or the fact that he drinks his tea noisily and lets it dribble down his chin or his habit of picking his nose are examples of behaviour which appear to be of minor importance to an outsider but can become intolerable to someone who has to observe them every day.

In some cases all that is required is for the old person to be told that his behaviour is offensive but it may be impossible for a child to do this, for reasons which have been discussed earlier, and professional intervention may be necessary to help the relatives say what they feel about the old person's behaviour.

If it proves impossible to cure the behaviour problem it is important to offer the relatives adequate relief by arranging for the old person to attend a day centre or day hospital or by arranging regular admissions of short duration.

Housing and financial problems

Caring for a disabled elderly relative at home can have financial consequences which cause problems, particularly for low-income families. It is important that they claim the Dependent Relative Allowance when filling in their Income Tax Return and that they are advised about the Attendance Allowance. This Allowance which is described in the Department of Health leaflet NI205 is for people who require 'frequent attention . . . in connection with . . . bodily functions or continual supervision in order to avoid substantial danger' to themselves or others. The Allowance is granted only after these criteria have been fulfilled for six months and is paid at two rates. The lower rate is paid if attendance is required during either the day or the night, and the higher rate is paid if the person needs attendance both day and night. If the lower rate is granted initially the person can apply to have their case reconsidered if he thinks that he needs help day and night. An appeal can be made against any decision which is felt to be wrong. The claim form, which is attached to leaflet NI205, can be completed by the disabled person or by someone else acting on his behalf (Gray and MacKenzie 1979).

The other important benefit is the Invalid Care Allowance (DHSS leaflet NI 212). This is payable to people who are 'not gainfully employed' and who are 'regularly and substantially engaged in caring for a severely disabled person' and the definition of 'severely disabled' is that the person should be in receipt of the Attendance Allowance at either the higher or the lower rate, or the Constant Attendance Allowance which is paid to disabled war pensioners or people disabled by an industrial disease. The Invalid Care Allowance is below 'the poverty line', that is it is less than the basic level of income defined by Social Security as necessary for subsistence and the carer may have to apply for a Supplementary Allowance to bring her income up to the subsistence level. However, the granting of an Invalid Care Allowance has one considerable benefit which the carer would otherwise not receive – she is credited with a Class I National Insurance contribution as though she were working. If an old person who is being looked after by a daughter who lives with, and is maintained by, that old person he may claim the Daughter's Services Allowance from the Inland Revenue.

In addition to these benefits relatives may be eligible for:
Free prescriptions (leaflet PC 11).
Reduced charges for dental treatment (leaflet F 11).
Reduced charges for glasses (leaflet F 11).
Help with rent and rates.

The common housing problems which occur when an elderly person is living with relatives are overcrowding and the inconvenience resulting from the elder's inability to reach the toilet. There are, unfortunately, no grants available to build granny-flats on to existing dwellings and overcrowding is difficult to relieve except for council tenants for it is usually possible to arrange for their rehousing in a larger dwelling by writing to the Community Physician. If the person is unable to reach the toilet it may be possible to adapt the dwelling, perhaps by building on a downstairs toilet which gives the old person independence and removes the need for a commode in a room used by other members of the family. The Domiciliary Occupational Therapist should also be consulted.

Help for single daughters

The National Council for the Single Woman and her Dependants, 29 Chilworth Mews, London W2, is a source of advice and support for single daughters wherever they live. There are now branches of this pressure group and advisory service in many parts of the country but if there is no local branch the head office can give invaluable advice and support directly to the single daughter.

9 Common handicaps

The distinction between disability and handicap has already been discussed (see p. 8). Disabilities are the functional limitations caused by disease, for example muscle weakness or joint stiffness, whereas handicaps are the social consequences, such as difficulties with self care and housework (Blaxter 1976).

THE ASSESSMENT OF DISABILITY (see p. 8)

The assessment of a person's disability obviously involves a clinical review of the causal disease but the psychological and social aspects of disability also have to be assessed. These are obviously unique to the individual who has a disability, but they can usefully be considered under four headings:
1. The person's personality before the onset of the disabling disease.
2. Her emotional response to her disability.
3. Her expectations.
4. The attitudes and expectations of other people.

Previous personality

Psychological tests which can measure various aspects of personality are available but they are primarily of use only to clinical psychologists: a general practitioner can obtain more reliable information by asking the patient questions about his outlook on life. If the patient was not well known before the onset of disability it may be useful to complement the patient's opinion with the opinion of relatives by asking questions such as 'What was his outlook on life – was he generally optimistic and hopeful or pessimistic?'; 'How did he react to adversity – was he easily discouraged or was he a fighter?'.

Practical implications

An appreciation of the patient's personality is not only helpful in planning rehabilitation. A change in the personality following the onset of a disabling disease suggests that some emotional reaction to the disability is unresolved.

Emotional responses

Each individual responds in his own way to disability but the reactions may be considered under four headings. Each of the four types of response causes a particular type of problem for the doctor who is trying to rehabilitate the disabled person (Table 9.1).

These responses are not four distinct conditions. A person may respond in all

The assessment of disability 157

Table 9.1.

Emotional response	Implications for rehabilitation
Depression	The depressed person may be too poorly motivated to agree on goals or to work towards them. He will also be very discouraged by failures
Anxiety	The anxious person may be unwilling to walk unaided or be left alone: he may be unwilling to accept goals set by the doctor because they introduce further uncertainty in his life
Bitterness	The person who is bitter often has a negative, pessimistic approach and an angry and hostile attitude to professional helpers and relatives
Denial	This may result in an unrealistically cheerful and optimistic 'I'm very happy with my lot' attitude, which may make the person refuse to accept that he could be fitter or more independent

four ways and the response may vary from day to day. The person may express one type of feeling to one person and another to someone else.

Practical implications

Rather than trying to classify the old person into one of the four boxes it is much better to create the opportunities for the disabled person to talk about her feelings; for example, 'Some people are puzzled by the fact that they are suffering while other people are spared – does that bother you at all? Do you ever feel bitter about it?' (see p. 115).

Attitudes and expectations of disabled old people

A disabled person may be poorly motivated to try to become independent because he is unconsciously unwilling to do anything which might lose him the advantage of being independent (see p. 196). There are, however, other reasons why some old people refuse to help themselves, which are less to do with a fear of isolation and more to do with their expectation that 'old people should be looked after'. There are two common reasons for this attitude.

The statement 'You are paid to do it' expresses the first reason, and the fact that older people pay for home help makes some believe, understandably perhaps, that they should determine what the home help should do. Similarly, the fact that a resident is paying to stay in an old people's home may make her demand that staff do everything for her. Again this is understandable because the old person may be paying about twice as much as she paid for the best holiday she ever had.

This attitude is hardened, in some old people, because they feel bitter that they are being forced to pay from their pension or savings, or from the sale of their house, when they know that other residents are 'paying nothing'. This is a source of considerable bitterness – 'It's very depressing, in fact it makes you sick. You save and save and then they say you have to pay £90 to stay in this home. If I had spent all my money on drink I would get the same food and everything' – and may produce resistance to the suggestion that the old person could do more to help herself. This is less of a problem for health workers, partly because old people do not pay for services in the same way, partly because the expectations of elderly people about 'care' are different from their expectations about 'treatment', but old people in hospital sometimes adopt a similar approach, saying – 'I've paid my rates and taxes and have a right to be looked after'.

The statement 'I've worked hard all my days' expresses the second reason and some old people are resistant to active forms of intervention such as physiotherapy or the encouragement of self help – 'Just let me be, I just want to die', and 'I'm too tired to do these tricks' are not uncommon responses and it must be accepted that many old people find the activities of everday life trying enough without taking on new tasks, as J. B. Priestley wrote in his autobiography *Instead of the Trees* (see p. 118).

This can raise very difficult ethical issues. How much pressure should be put on an old person who is not well motivated, who refuses to go to day hospital for instance, or who refuses to do at home what she can do in the physiotherapy department? The combination of a disabling disease, loss of fitness, and depression is very powerful and the problems faced by elderly disabled people are considerable. By reducing the symptoms of disease and by inspiring hope and confidence it is often possible to help an older patient overcome these problems but the right to refuse what we see as 'help' but what the old person sees as 'interference' has to be recognized.

Practical implications

It is essential to be aware of these attitudes and sympathetic towards them, even though an old person appears unco-operative because of them. The point to make to all old people is that of the encouragement of self help and activity is principally for their benefit and not just to relieve busy and harrassed staff or relatives. It is sometimes necessary to be frank and to tell an old person who is reluctant to exert herself that she is unlikely to die easily and gently if she does nothing for herself, as some old people believe, but that she will probably become immobile, incontinent, and uncomfortable long before she dies.

Attitudes and expectations of other people

'If I buy a wheelchair will you push my mother in it like all the other residents?'

'Would you like us to organize a jumble sale to buy wheelchairs for all the residents?'

Many people are over-protective about old people, as these quotes illustrate, and there is considerable resistance to an active approach which encourages independence and self help. Such an approach is seen as 'cruel' and 'callous'.

The reasons for this attitude, and the expectations which result from it, vary from one person to another, but there are two common reasons. One is ignorance, for many people are ignorant of the fact that many of the problems of old people are preventable and treatable. The second is guilt, because many members of the public and relatives are aware that they could do more than they are doing, and feel guilty that they are not. Their means of coping with their guilt is to demand that old people be 'cared for', which often means that they should be spared all discomfort and risk (see p. 120).

Mr. T. was still able to get the bus to his club for a drink once or twice a week, but every time he went to get the bus a member of the public came into the home to 'report' that there was a resident on the street and to criticize staff for allowing him to be 'at risk'.

Practical implications

When someone reacts in a hostile or angry manner to an old person's attempts to be independent or to the encouragement of a nurse or physiotherapist that he should try to overcome his disabilities, it is important to try to understand why he is reacting in such a way, and not to react angrily in turn. It is, however, often possible to guess how other people may react to an attempt to encourage independence and it is useful to ask the question, 'I wonder what Mr S's son and daughter-in-law will say if they see him struggling to cook for himself?' and to open a discussion with the old person's relatives to explain the reasons why he is being allowed to struggle instead of being 'helped' by having other people perform every task for him.

Relatives often need to be educated about the need to let a disabled person struggle to achieve something to prevent unfitness and dependence (Fig. 9.1).

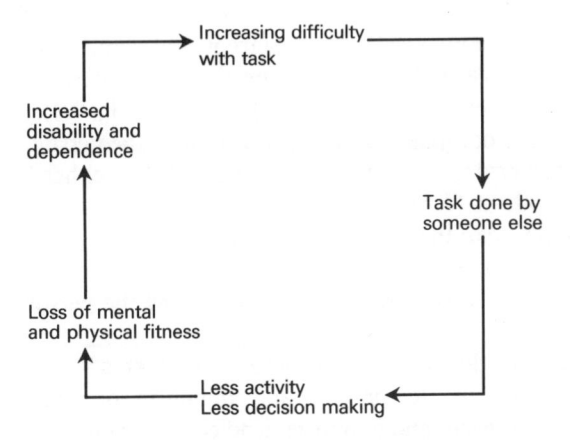

Fig. 9.1. The vicious cycle of dependency

> **Useful advice for old people and their relatives**
>
> *Guidelines for helping disabled people*
>
> 1. Remember that the physiotherapy and occupational therapy of everyday life is of vital importance in old age (see p. 132). The muscles, joints, and nerves used in making tea and toast are the same as those used in dressing and undressing and the decisions involved in making a stew or in running a household budget are of vital importance in preserving mental fitness.
> 2. Be careful not to take on more and more tasks because it is quicker for you to do them or because you don't like to see him struggling or because you are afraid he will injure himself.
> 3. Be careful that his gratitude does not influence you to do more than is necessary to earn more gratitude.
> 4. Try to arrange any task which you have to perform so that the handicapped person is able to contribute to its completion.

THE CONTRIBUTION OF PHYSIOTHERAPY AND OCCUPATIONAL THERAPY

The loss of ability which results from the disabling disease has serious physical and psychological consequences (Fig. 9.2).

The objective of the physiotherapist is to prevent or minimize the secondary effects of disease – joint stiffness, muscle weakness, and loss of confidence. Although she is depicted at stage 5 in the handicap algorithm she should, wherever possible, be involved from the start of treatment. This is, unfortunately, rarely possible in general practice owing to the inadequate development of community or 'direct access' physiotherapy services (Fig. 9.3).

The task of the occupational therapist is to help the person with a disability to adapt to her environment so well that she will be neither handicapped nor dependent on others. Her approach is in three stages.

1. Education – can the person learn new ways of doing everyday tasks that minimize the effects of her disability?

2. Aids – can aids to daily living ('ADL') allow the person to regain independence?

3. Adaptation – does her dwelling need to be adapted?

Physiotherapists try to prevent and minimize disability. Occupational therapists try to prevent and minimize handicap. Obviously there is an overlap between the function of occupational and physiotherapists but the domiciliary

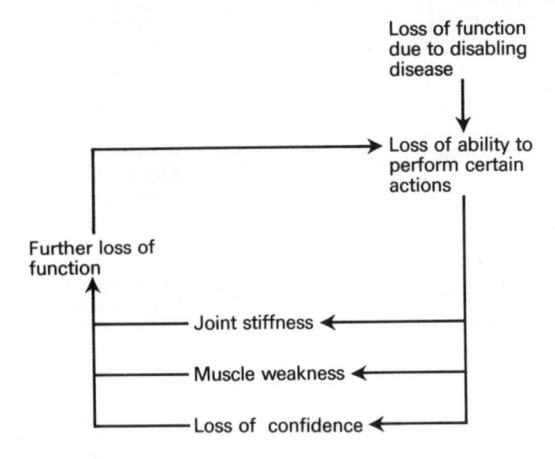

Fig. 9.2. The vicious cycle of disability.

occupational therapist is usually more involved in helping people with disabilities who are in their own homes because a higher proportion of 'OTs' work outside hospital in Social Services Departments as domiciliary occupational therapists.

IDENTIFYING HANDICAPPED PATIENTS

The common handicaps in old age are problems with self-care and the interruption of a normal social life which results from immobility. A disabled old person may have difficulty with one or more of the following list of tasks.

Dressing and undressing.
Washing all over.
Reaching the toilet in time.
Being able to use the toilet cleanly and safely.
Getting enough to eat and drink.
Doing light housework.
Doing light gardening.
Getting out to see relatives and friends or to visit the pub or church.

If one handicap is present one or more of the others may also be presented and a checklist such as this chould be used when one type of handicap has been identified.

These are the common handicaps and they are obvious problems but their identification may be difficult because they may not be brought to the general

162 Common handicaps

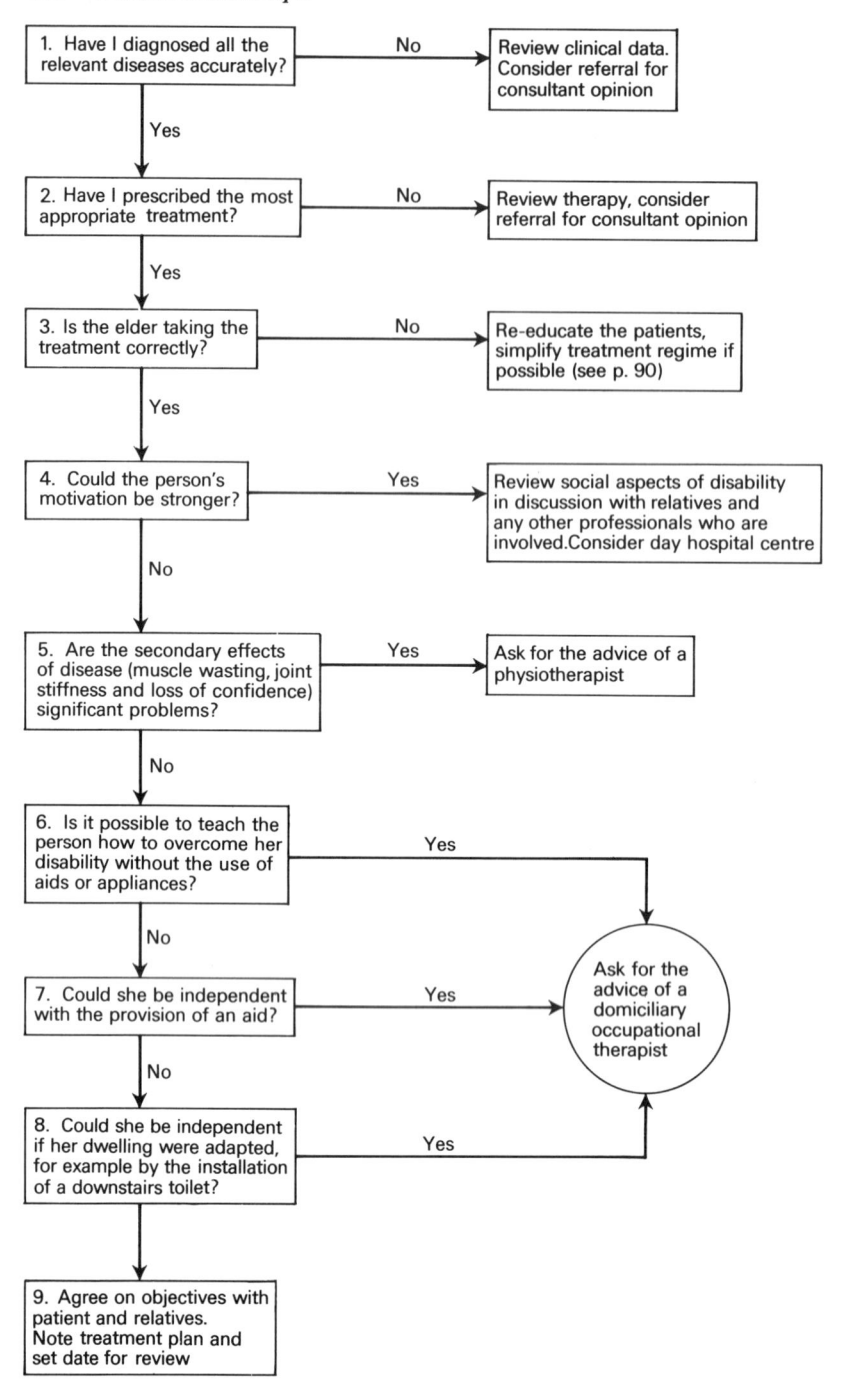

```
1. Have I diagnosed all the relevant diseases accurately?
  — No → Review clinical data. Consider referral for consultant opinion
  — Yes ↓

2. Have I prescribed the most appropriate treatment?
  — No → Review therapy, consider referral for consultant opinion
  — Yes ↓

3. Is the elder taking the treatment correctly?
  — No → Re-educate the patients, simplify treatment regime if possible (see p. 90)
  — Yes ↓

4. Could the person's motivation be stronger?
  — Yes → Review social aspects of disability in discussion with relatives and any other professionals who are involved. Consider day hospital centre
  — No ↓

5. Are the secondary effects of disease (muscle wasting, joint stiffness and loss of confidence) significant problems?
  — Yes → Ask for the advice of a physiotherapist
  — No ↓

6. Is it possible to teach the person how to overcome her disability without the use of aids or appliances?
  — Yes → Ask for the advice of a domiciliary occupational therapist
  — No ↓

7. Could she be independent with the provision of an aid?
  — Yes → Ask for the advice of a domiciliary occupational therapist
  — No ↓

8. Could she be independent if her dwelling were adapted, for example by the installation of a downstairs toilet?
  — Yes → Ask for the advice of a domiciliary occupational therapist
  ↓

9. Agree on objectives with patient and relatives. Note treatment plan and set date for review
```

Fig. 9.3. The handicap algorithm.

practitioner's attention. In some cases they are. An old person or her relatives may seek the general practitioner's advice because she is handicapped in one or more of the ways listed but in many cases medical help is not sought. The reason for this is that handicaps, like other symptoms of disease in old age, are often assumed to be the inevitable consequences of the untreatable ageing process and are not seen as the potentially curable results of disease. If the old person or her relatives are of this opinion then they may not 'bother' the general practitioner. Instead they seek help directly from the services which can perform the task for the old person rather than from the services which can help the elder regain the ability to perform them for herself, namely the services of the general practitioner. Thus handicaps are often referred directly to the meals-on-wheels service, or the home help service, or an old people's home without first consulting the general practitioner to see if he can reduce the old person's degree of disability.

Obviously it is impossible for the general practitioner to assess every referral to all the social services. There is, however, one type of referral for a social service which the general practitioner should investigate carefully – referral for residential care (see p. 106).

COPING WITH COMMON HANDICAPS

Having reduced the patient's disability to its lowest possible level by (i) review of diagnosis, treatment, and compliance; (ii) physiotherapy to prevent joint stiffness, muscle weakness; and loss of confidence; and (iii) reviewing the psychological aspects of disability it is appropriate to try to help patients to cope with the residual level of disability. It is also necessary to help relatives cope with the burden which the old person's dependence places on them because members of the family provide most of the help for people with disabilities (Table 9.2).

Furthermore relatives may not seek for help even though they are finding the burden of providing help a strain and for this reason questions about the help

Table 9.2.

Sources of help given to elderly people who can bath only with help

Help received from	Percentage
Person(s) in household	61.0
Relative(s) outside, usually children or 'children-in-law'	18.5
Friend(s) outside household	4.7
District nurse	8.7
Home help	1.6
Other person	3.5
No-one	2.0
Not stated	2.4

From Hunt, A. (1978). *The elderly at home*, p. 75. HMSO, London.

given to disabled relatives should be included in a case-finding approach to family problems (see p. 147) and any families who are supporting a disabled elder should be included in any screening programmes.

When advising relatives it is useful to try to teach them how to help the old person use her own abilities in the first place, then to suggest that some aids might be helpful, and finally to consider whether or not the dwelling needs to be adapted. The involvement of the domiciliary occupational therapist is essential if the dwelling is to be adapted and she should also be involved if aids are required, although old people and their relatives are often able to devise simple aids and adapt ordinary household equipment to suit the limitations of the person who is disabled.

Dressing and undressing

Dressing problems can contribute to:
  Dependence on relatives which leads to depression.
  Hypothermia.
  'Incontinence' due to inability to undress in time when at the toilet.
  Falls.

Useful advice for old people and their relatives

Dressing and undressing

It is important not to help a disabled person with all aspects of dressing or undressing but only with those parts which he finds most difficult. The best plan is to give him enough time to dress and only help with the action which is most difficult – for example, putting the second arm in a jacket or pulling up trousers. Some people, not surprisingly, become embarrassed or flustered with someone standing over them waiting to help and may ask for more help than is necessary because of this. It is, therefore, usually wise to leave the person to dress saying 'call me when you need a hand'.

Relatives should be told about the dangers of doing too much for the disabled person. They should be told about the types of dressing aids and special clothes which are available and encouraged to discuss difficulties with the district nurse or domiciliary occupational therapist if in difficulty. This is commonly the case with patients who have had a stroke.

Washing all over

Enquiries about washing should be carefully worded because they can give offence. One way of approaching the subject is by asking about washing while asking about a whole range of other activities, for example by asking 'do you find that you are not so mobile as you were, do you feel as safe while using the bath as you did?' If the person says that they can no longer use the bath, he can be asked if he is able to wash all over. Remember that some disabled people do not bathe because they are too nervous of falling, although they are physically able to step in and out of the bath.

Sometimes the advice that an old person needs is that which is most difficult to give, namely the advice that it is becoming obvious that he is having difficulty bathing, either because he looks dirty or is smelling. Some old people have a poor sense of smell and do not notice odours which are strong to other people and even if an old person's sense of smell is good the change may take place so slowly that he may fail to notice that he is dirtier or smellier than he was a year ago. This is obviously a very sensitive subject but it is sometimes best to speak plainly and it is often easier for an outsider to do it than for a close relative to do so.

Useful advice for old people and their relatives

On bathing

If the old person is nervous it is often sufficient just to be in the house or near the door in case of need. If he is physically disabled, however, it is usually necessary to assist him.

It is important to encourage the person to move slowly and calmly, and not to be tense or grab you or the bath. Keep the person encouraged by talking to him, praising his successes, advising him to 'take a rest and five deep breaths' when he has completed one stage successfully, and don't be afraid to use that invaluable aid – humour.

All old people should use a non-slip bath mat.

Do not spend any money on rails or a shower without asking the advice of the domiciliary occupational therapist.

If the old person becomes too nervous to bath even with someone to help the advice of the district nurse or domiciliary occupational therapist should be sought.

If your back gets painful when helping your relative to bath ask for help.

Relatives should be given all this advice, but it must be remembered that the most difficult problem for relatives may be embarrassment and it may be appropriate to encourage a son or daughter to ask for help with bathing even though they are physically capable of helping.

Doing light housework and gardening

Failure to manage the upkeep of home and garden can cause or contribute to
Depression and hopelessness.
Dependence on relatives.
Hypothermia.
Falls.

Sometimes the old person can be given advice about how to do her housework more easily but may need aids such as a tap turner or a long-handled dustpan. Similarly in gardening, the use of long-handled clippers may allow a person to trim the edges of the lawn again.

Adaptations

The house may need to be adapted to make housework easier, perhaps by putting in a gas fire, although the benefits of a coal fire should not be underestimated, or by installing an efficient hot water system. In addition the garden can be adapted, although there are no financial grants available for this. Shrubs can be put in to cover the ground, part of the grass can be paved or, best of all, flower beds can be raised to allow the person to manage independently.

Useful advice for old people and their relatives

On housework and gardening

Remember that housework is very beneficial for elderly people; it provides useful physio- and occupational therapy.

The best way of helping is to divide the tasks which have to be done into parts which can be done by the old person and parts which have to be done by someone else, to allow the old person to participate as much as possible.

Try to allow the old person to make as many decisions as possible even though she is not able to do all the work.

Ask the advice of the domiciliary occupational therapist if the old person is unable to do any housework or is having increasing difficulty.

Getting enough to eat and drink

Relatives are often worried that an old person is not getting enough to eat or drink and request meals on wheels or the services of a home help. However, before providing food for the old person it is important to determine whether or not the old person has a nutritional problem and to identify the precise

Table 9.3.

Reason for difficulty with eating and drinking	Possible solution

Ignorance	More common among widowers but some elderly women are also ignorant of the most important foods to eat when they are eating less than when younger and more active.
	    Attendance at cookery class in day centre.
	    Provision for health education leaflets or a book such as *Easy eating for one or two* by Louise Davies.
	    Referral to geriatric hospital for advice from dietician for difficult cases

Inability to reach shops	Review mobility problems (see p. 45) Arrange for help with shopping perhaps by volunteer (see p. 168)
Difficulty with preparation and cooking	Review medical reason for difficulty which may be immobility, hand weakness, visual failure, co-ordination problems, or inability to stand for a long time. The advice of the domiciliary OT is very useful for such problems. If mobility is the main reason it should be possible to provide everything an old person needs for twenty-four hours within reach of her chair by intelligent use of Thermos flasks and plastic containers

Difficulty with eating	Check dentures
	    Review reason for difficulty, commonly hand weakness, visual failure or co-ordination problems following stroke.
	    Refer to domiciliary OT for provision of aids

Inadequate motivation	The appetite may be impaired when the following conditions prevail:
	    Isolation (see p. 195)
	    Dementia
	    Depression
	    Alcohol abuse
	    Drug side-effects
	    Chronic pain
	The solution to this problem is the solution of the causal problem but attendance at a lunch club is often more effective than meals on wheels no matter what the reason for the loss of appetite

reason why the old person is having difficulty and to provide a solution which gives the elder as much independence as possible (Table 9.3).

HELP FOR HANDICAPPED PEOPLE

Home helps and organizers

The job of the home help is to help disabled elderly people to live at home. They do this by helping them with their housework and with shopping and food preparation – at least that is the physical component of their work but in many cases it is the psychological help and support which is just as important as, or even more important than, the practical help.

Often the home help and client develop feelings of warm personal affection for one another. This close relationship is obviously not without its dangers. The old person may become dependent on the helper and the home help may become closely emotionally involved with the elder. However, the drawbacks are almost always outweighed by the benefits because it is often the moral support of a home help which gives an old person the necessary motivation to struggle at home.

In most social services departments home helps are not encouraged to perform personal care, that is to bathe an old person or to undress her and help her to bed, but home helps often do much more than is their job description and give personal care. This has been recognized and in an increasing number of departments certain home helps, who may be called home care assistants, are trained to perform tasks which were once the sole responsibility of the nursing auxiliary.

The amount of home help which a home help organizer can allocate an elderly person influenced by many factors, notably by the availability of home help staff and the needs of other clients. However, it is not unreasonable for a general practitioner to expect of the home help service that his patient be given help on all seven dys of the week before she is deemed to be in need of residential care (see p. 106). In some areas it is now possible for an old person to be allocated two or even three daily visits by a home help but it is often necessary for the home help organizer to arrange for this seven day cover by the use of voluntary help or paid 'good neighbours' who undertake to perform simple tasks such as meal preparation at weekends. The organizer has to juggle with her resources to try to meet all the needs in the population for which she is responsible but she is much more than a director of labour. She has to recruit home helps, prepare them for work and support them in their difficult task. Frequently the organizer's problem is to stop the home help doing too much or becoming over-involved rather than the usual manager's problem of trying to stimulate the workforce to do more.

Volunteers

Because the skills and expectations of volunteers vary so widely it is important to learn what the local voluntary groups have to offer rather than relying on assumptions based on previous experience in another area. It is usually easy to find out which groups are active in the area covered by the practice and to ask a representative to come along to a practice meeting or working lunch to speak about the contribution their group has to offer and, even more important, what types of problems its members are reluctant, or are not prepared, to tackle. It is sometimes assumed that volunteers will tackle anything which does not fit into the job descriptions of professional workers but this is not the case. Each organization has its own set of rules but there are two types of tasks which are usually regarded as inappropriate by the organizers of voluntary organizations and by the volunteers themselves.

Firstly, many volunteers are reluctant to tackle tasks which involve touching the person other than on the hand or arm. In British society large areas of the body are taboo, untouchable except by one's marital partners or by a professional such as a doctor or nurse. Similarly the naked body embarrasses many people and it is therefore inappropriate to expect volunteers to bathe an elderly person or help her to dress or undress or to deal with her incontinence. Members of St. John's or Red Cross groups may be willing to undertake this type of work in emergency, for example when the old person's relatives have gone away on holiday, but the members of most other groups are usually unwilling to touch people or to help them when naked.

Secondly, tasks which involve regular, open-ended commitment are viewed with apprehension by most volunteers. It is not that volunteers are frightened of hard work but many are afraid of the dependence which long-term involvement may foster. It is not uncommon for a volunteer to regard the old person who has been referred as someone who will deteriorate and eventually become so dependent that the volunteer will be unable to go away for a holiday or even a weekend. This degree of dependence is not unusual and many volunteers have heard of other voluntary helpers who have been 'caught' or 'trapped' and who have not been supported by the professionals when problems developed. Of course many volunteers do support old people regularly for years but it is usually more appropriate to request involvement for only a limited period of time in the first instance rather than asking for an open-ended commitment.

Using volunteers

The types of problem volunteers tackle willingly and well greatly outnumber those which they are reluctant to accept.

1. Visits and support in emergencies: it is often difficult, and sometimes impossible, to mobilize the home help service or visits from a nursing auxiliary in the evenings or at weekends when an old person has suffered an incapacitating injury, such as Colles' fracture or when his principal supporter has herself been taken ill. Volunteers are usually willing to provide short-term help, such as preparing meals, making tea, and checking that the old person is safe, until statutory services can be mobilized. A list of the telephone numbers of each of the contacts of the local voluntary groups such as churches, Red Cross, St. John's, Good Neighbour, Fish, WVRS, and Age Concern schemes, should be kept near the surgery phone.

2. Support and relief for relatives: volunteers can often provide someone to sit in with the old person thus allowing relatives to go out for an evening. Voluntary organizations may be able to provide enough help to allow relatives to go away for the weekend although the old person may need some persuasion to accept voluntary help. In addition the British Red Cross Society and the St. John Ambulance Association and Brigade both organize excellent home nursing courses for relatives.

3. Trips out of the home: these can prevent and alleviate depression and

confusion and visits to the church, pub, or club which the old person formerly attended can often be arranged with the transport provided by members of the church or club or pub regulars.

4. Relief of suffering through prayer: it is important that the church is not simply regarded as a provider of welfare services. Many elderly people find their suffering relieved or easier to bear if they can be given the opportunity to speak to and pray with a priest at home or, preferably, in a congregation.

5. The provision of funds: voluntary organizations are very useful for fundraising. Many old people do not like to be the direct recipients of such local charity and the general practitioner may be able to suggest to the local organizations ways of spending their money which benefit old people who are most in need. The purchase of electric blankets for district nurses to lend to people at risk of hypothermia, the payment of voluntary drivers or even equipment for the health centre are better ways of spending hard-earned money than the Christmas food parcel. Nevertheless, it is often very helpful to be able to raise £40 or £50 from a voluntary organization to help pay for a gas fire or some other expensive object.

There are a few principal sources of charitable funds but the sensitivity of many old people to 'charity' should always be remembered (Table 9.4).

Table 9.4.

Source	Means of making contact
Former regiment or regiment of dead husband	Find the name of the regiment or service in which the old person or her husband served and, if possible, the old person's regimental number. Then ask someone from the British Legion to visit
Former employer	Phone or write to the personnel department of firm or business
Local charities	Make application on old person's behalf to a local charity. Local Age Concern or Council for Voluntary Service should know of all relevant services
Relevant national charity	There are charities for many occupational groups. These are contained in the Charities Digest. The Citizens' Advice Bureau will be able to give information

Helping volunteers

General practitioners can be of great use to voluntary organizations. The general practitioner can help in the training of volunteers, or 'preparation' as some voluntary organizations call it in preference to the term 'training'. Offers of help, with the assurance that a fee is not expected, will be welcome as may be the offer of the health centre for an evening meeting.

10 Social problems

WHAT ARE THE SOCIAL PROBLEMS

The family doctor is normally a person's first point of contact with the health services and he may well be the first person through whom an approach is made to the social services.

Social problems and medical problems

The World Health Organization's definition of health – complete physical, mental, and social well being and not merely the absence of disease – has been much criticized but it has served a useful purpose in emphasizing that the physical, mental, and social aspects of an individual should always be considered. The fact that three aspects were stipulated might be thought to imply that there was some natural and clear distinction between physical, mental, and social wellbeing but it is obvious that they blend into one another and have been distinguished from one another artificially. Artificial though the distinction may be it is of great significance for the general practitioner and general hospital services, psychiatric services, and social services – and the general practitioner often has to involve all three for the benefit of his patient.

Social problems may have medical causes and medical problems may have social consequences (Fig 10.1).

There is therefore a need for comprehensive assessment. Obviously this cannot be done whenever a need for a social service such as meals on wheels is

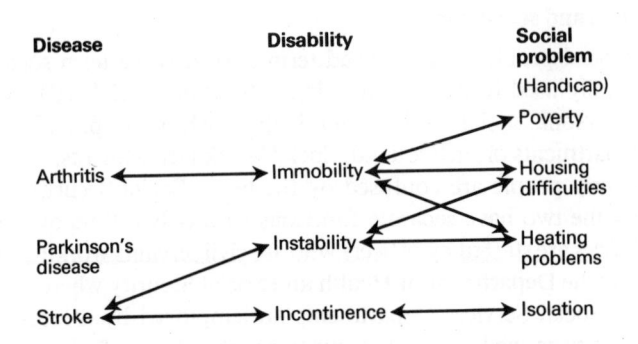

Disease	Disability	Social problem (Handicap)
Arthritis	Immobility	Poverty
Parkinson's disease	Instability	Housing difficulties
Stroke	Incontinence	Heating problems
		Isolation

Fig. 10.1. The radical–social problem continuum.

171

defined by the old person or her relatives, although the knowledge that someone has been referred for a social service should prompt two questions:
1. Why has she become unable to look after herself?
2. Is this due to normal aging or could it be the result of a treatable disease?

This is particularly important when an old person is said to be 'in need of residential care' by a relative or social worker. This opinion is usually based on the fact that the old person is handicapped and dependent on other people for basic tasks such as cooking or dressing. However, the decision to relinquish one's home and move into an old people's home is such a major decision that every attempt should be made to try to tackle her handicaps by reducing her level of disability rather than by increasing her dependence. One study of one hundred people referred for residential care showed that only 68 of them actually needed residential care. Eleven needed hospital care but fifteen were found not to need either hospital care nor a place in an old people's home (Table 10.1).

Table 10.1. *Result of comprehensive medial review of 100 people referred for residential care*

Outcome	No. of patients
Residential care	68
Sheltered housing	4
Long-term psychogeriatric care	5
Long-term geriatric care	5
Hospital treatment of tuberculosis	1
Remained at home because:	
Improvement	6
Managing with short-term hospital admissions to relieve relatives	2
Refused residential care	2
Moved to lodgings	1
Moved elsewhere	1
Died	5
	100

From Brocklehurst, J. C. *et al.* (1978). Medical screening of old people accepted for residential care. *Lancet ii*, 141–2.

Social services and social work

The term 'social problems' is a broad term and so is the term social services which is usually used to describe housing, education, social security, and the health and personal social services, that is those which are provided by Social Services Departments or, in Scotland, Social Work Departments.

Many elderly people are confused by the terms Social Security and Social Services but the two have separate functions with only a little overlap. Social Security Offices are staffed by officers who are civil servants working in a system controlled by the Department of Health and Social Security whereas those who work in the Social Services Departments are employed by a local authority, either the county council or, in cities, the borough. This confusion is not helped by the fact that the Secretary of State is the Secretary for Health and Social Services although he is responsible for the Department of Health and Social Security.

Social Services Departments have many functions but those which are of relevance to old people may be grouped under five headings.

1. Domiciliary services:
– home help;
– meals on wheels;
– lunch clubs and day centres, and the transport to reach them;
– aids to daily living and house alterations, and the provision of a domiciliary occupational therapy service;
– telephone installation and the payment of rental;
– the supply and licensing of radio and television sets;
– a laundry service for soiled linen.

These are only major services. Under the Chronically Sick and Disabled Persons Act of 1970 (The CSDP) a Department can, in theory, pay for almost any aid or service which will allow a disabled person to lead an independent life. In practice, however, it is only possible for the Department to do what it can afford and the services provided are limited by the resources made available to them. The CSDP also required each Department to keep a register of handicapped persons and any handicapped individual can apply for registration but it is not necessary to be registered to be eligible for any of these services. Many handicapped people are reluctant to have their names held on such a list and can be reassured that they will not be refused services because they refuse to register.

2. Support of, and co-operation with, voluntary organizations.

3. The provision of information, not only about its own services but about housing, financial, and legal services. The local Age Concern office is another very useful source of information and the old person can be encouraged to enquire there if he is reluctant to approach 'the Welfare'. The Citizens' Advice Bureau is another useful source of advice, and is particularly useful with respect to legal or housing problems. In some areas there are also specialist Housing Advice Centres which work closely with the CAB.

4. The provision of residential accommodation (see p. 187) and the supervision of private and voluntary old people's homes.

5. The employment of social workers, which is the function which many people find most difficult to understand because the job of the social worker is not easy to describe. Part of the job relates to the other functions of the department. The social worker is the person who provides the information and who works with voluntary services and he is also the person who is responsible for assessing the need for services such as telephones and residential care in old people's homes. (The staff of old people's homes are also social workers, termed residential social workers, whereas those who work in the community

are sometimes referred to as field social workers but are usually just called 'social workers').

In assessing the need for services the social worker has to serve several different functions. He sometimes has to act as agent for the old person, helping her fill out forms and make phone calls; he may have to act as her advocate and argue his client's need for a place in a home in competition with the claims of other social workers for their clients; and he may have to act as a rationer of scarce resources and decide which individual is in greatest need. However, the social worker is not just a trader – acting as an agent, putting in bids or deciding on the best bid – he does not only become concerned with the old person after the decision to enter a home has been made but is concerned with the manner in which that decision is reached, in helping the old person evaluate all the options, resisting undue pressure from other people, and reaching a decision which is the best for them.

Social workers have a role which is unrelated to functions of their department or team. They are not just employed to ensure that the social services are effectively and efficiently provided, and the part which the social worker plays in helping an old person reach a decision about residential care illustrates this. The objectives of social work are to help individuals and families to appreciate those aspects of their problems which result from their own attitudes and values, and from their attitudes towards, and feelings about, one another, and to help the individual or family change so that their problems are reduced (Brearley 1975, 1978) (see p. 102).

Inappropriate referrals

It is useful at this stage to list some of the types of problems which would be considered by most social workers as being of too low priority to accept.

1. Referrals of lonely old people 'for visiting', although a referral to social services for attendance at a day centre is appropriate.
2. Housing problems which should be referred to the housing department or to Age Concern, Citizens' Advice Bureau, or a Housing Aid Centre.
3. Financial problems which should be referred to Social Security or to Age Concern or the Citizens' Advice Bureau (see p. 104).

COMMON SOCIAL PROBLEMS AND THE GENERAL PRACTITIONER

The remainder of this chapter will be concerned with the common social problems as identified by old people.

Housing problems.
Financial problems.
Heating problems.
Isolation.

To solve a social problem an old person has to take four steps (Fig. 10.2).

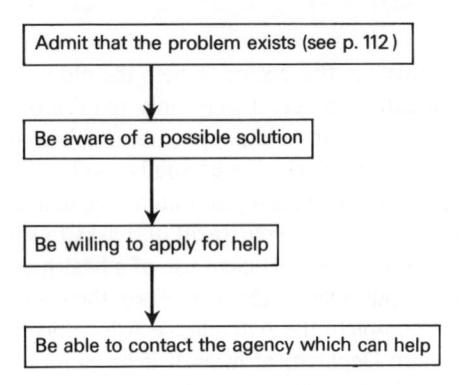

```
┌─────────────────────────────────────────┐
│ Admit that the problem exists (see p. 112) │
└─────────────────────────────────────────┘
                    │
                    ▼
┌─────────────────────────────────┐
│ Be aware of a possible solution │
└─────────────────────────────────┘
                    │
                    ▼
┌─────────────────────────────┐
│ Be willing to apply for help │
└─────────────────────────────┘
                    │
                    ▼
┌──────────────────────────────────────────┐
│ Be able to contact the agency which can help │
└──────────────────────────────────────────┘
```

Fig. 10.2. The four steps to help.

The general practitioner can help an old person take each of these steps even though he does not have a detailed knowledge of the full range of social and voluntary services which are available.

Facilitating the admission of problems

The GP may be the most trusted of the professionals visiting the old person and she may therefore be willing to admit to him that she has a social problem although denying its existence to relatives and other professionals.

If the old person is not well known to the GP it may facilitate her admission of her difficulties and allay her fears that she will be institutionalized if the doctor states explicitly that he believes that the best course of action is for her to stay in her own home before asking about any difficulties which she may be having (see p. 119).

Informing about services

The doctor need not know all the details of all the services but he should be aware of the more important benefits and services which are available and, equally important, know about the other professionals such as the environmental health officer, and advisory services such as Age Concern, who can give specialized advice.

Encouraging application

Many old people are reluctant to apply for any help because they fear that they will be humiliated, or patronized, or subjected to a distressing investigation. Many still fear the Poor Law which no longer exists. They need to be told that many of the benefits and services available do not entail a means test and reassured that most officials are sympathetic and sensitive when carrying out a means test. Many are reluctant to accept what they consider 'charity' and need to be encouraged to think of the services which are available as a right, not as a charity offered by do-gooders.

Making the link

Finally it may be necessary for the doctor to help the old person make the link with the agency which can help her: it may only require one phone call or a short note to obtain help but many old people are unable to make a phone call or to write a short note. Social workers are usually too busy to pay home visits just to help an old person fill out a form, although they will often help if an old person goes to the Social Services Department and asks to speak to the officer on duty, and it is not making a very efficient use of a health visitor's time to ask her to visit solely for this purpose. Often, therefore, the simplest step is for the general practitioner to complete the Attendance Allowance form or to phone the Environmental Health Department himself if he cannot find a neighbour, relative, or friend who is sufficiently trusted by the old person to be able to be asked to make the necessary link.

POVERTY

People are poverty stricken when their income, even if it is adequate for survival, falls markedly below that of the community. Then they cannot have what the larger community regards as the minimum necessary for decency and they cannot wholly escape, therefore, the judgements of the larger community that they are indecent. They are degraded, for in the literal sense they live outside the grades or categories which the community regards as acceptable.

John Kenneth Galbraith

Absolute and relative poverty

It is useful to distinguish between these two types of poverty. Absolute poverty refers to the difference between the real value of the person's income and the prices of essential commodities; those who live below the poverty line are in absolute poverty and have difficulty in purchasing the necessities of life. Relative poverty referrs to the difference between a person's income and the average levels of income in the community in which he lives. In relative terms elderly people are impoverished for their income is much lower than the average wage and the relative poverty is greater the older the age group considered. The average income of older groups of old people is lower than that of younger age groups, partly because fewer have occupational pensions but also because of the higher proportion of women, for single women have, on average, the lowest income.

Relative poverty symbolizes and perpetuates the low status of elderly people and contributes to their feelings of worthlessness and their low self-esteeem but is it not so marked as it was because the net income of a pensioner which was 34 per cent of the net average industrial wage in 1948 had risen to 51 per cent by 1978. The absolute poverty of elderly people has been more markedly reduced for the value of the old age pension with respect to prices doubled between 1948 and 1978. There is little that an individual doctor can do to reduce the extent of relative poverty for that is a problem which requires social and political action but he can help an old person come to terms with feelings of worthlessness and depression which may be caused or aggravated by her low income. He can also help prevent and cure absolute poverty by helping her to maximize her income.

Delusions of poverty

Some elderly people accept their poverty too easily and have to be encouraged to apply for help (see p. 116). There are others, however, who hold the opposite attitude and believe that their financial position is much worse than is actually the case. Some do not alter their life style but become very parsimonious and count every penny, which can lead to problems if they become forgetful because they may accuse the home help or the warden of theft. A small proportion become obsessively concerned with money and refuse to heat their dwellings or to spend an adequate amount on food, or clothes, or the maintenance and repair of their dwellings.

There are a number of possible reasons for this and usually more than one is present.
- Some old people think that debt is shameful.
- Some associate debt with compulsory admission to the 'Workhouse'.
- Some housebound old people have been confused by decimalization and inflation and find the price of goods frighteningly high – 'twelve shillings for a dozen eggs? You can take them back.'

It is possible to prevent delusions of poverty if isolation is prevented and if the old person is helped and encouraged to retain full control of her affairs. If they develop they are often difficult to dispel. It may be possible to modify the elder's behaviour if the general practitioner is prepared to take a firm old-fashioned 'doctor's orders' approach but the solution is rarely as simple as this and it is better to attempt to re-educate the elderly person about the true value of her pension. The home help can play a vital part in this and the advice of a domiciliary occupational therapist can also be useful. If problems are very severe it may be necessary to appoint someone to manage the elder's affairs by application to the Court of Protection.

SOCIAL SECURITY

The Social Security system is extremely complex but the benefits for which elderly people are eligible can be considered under four main headings:

1. National Insurance benefits which are paid to those who have paid sufficient contributions – Retirement Pensions – or the widows of those who have paid sufficient contributions – Widows' Pensions.

2. Non-contributory benefits which are paid to those whose income falls below the poverty line even though they have not contributed to the National Insurance scheme. Supplementary pensions and rent and rate rebates are the

main non-contributory benefits. The over-80s pension is also a non-contributory pension granted solely on the grounds of age.

3. War Pensions.

4. Allowances granted to people solely on the grounds that they are severely disabled – the Attendance Allowance and the Invalid Care Allowance.

National Insurance Benefits

The retirement pension is paid to those who have reached retirement age provided that they have paid sufficient National Insurance contributions during their working life. It is not paid to those whose income comes above a certain level. This rule is known as 'the earnings rule' but it does not apply to men aged over 70 or women aged over 65, who can earn as much as they wish and still claim their retirement pension. There is a leaflet entitled 'Your Retirement Pension' (leaflet NP32) which gives all the necessary details. The widows of retirement pensioners also receive a national insurance pension.

In general the National Insurance system works smoothly and the general practitioner need not concern himself about whether or not the old person is claiming the retirement or widow's pension because it is paid automatically even if she does not make a claim. However, the level at which the retirement and widow's pension is set is actually just below the official poverty line set by the Government. Therefore, if the old person's only income is a retirement or widow's pension he or she should also apply for a supplementary pension which will be described below.

Those who are in receipt of a retirement or widow's pension may be eligible for help with rent or rates and they may still be eligible even though they have income from other sources and are well above the poverty line. Therefore all elderly people except those who are obviously wealthy should be encouraged to apply for financial assistance with their housing costs (see p. 185).

Non-contributory benefits

Supplementary pensions

This pension is granted to any old person whose income falls below the poverty line even if they have not paid National Insurance contributions. The old person may refer to this pension as 'National Assistance' which was its name until 1966, or refer to it simply as 'my social security' whereas the retirement pension is often referred to as 'my old age pension', although it is, of course, also part of Social Security.

Before the pension is granted the old person has to declare her income and, which may be even more difficult, her savings and this declaration and the questions which the social security officer may have to ask is what is known as the means test. The social security office staff work out the person's needs by adding rent and rates and any mortgage interest to the amount of money which is set as the income necessary for essential items by the Government of the day, and calculate the difference between the person's income and her needs. This is the amount paid as supplementary pension.

The means test can be very upsetting and most elderly people know about the means test, having heard gossip and rumours. Unfortunately, the image is offputting and many old people will not apply for supplementary pension because of their image of prying and censorious officials challenging their statements and hinting that they are being deceitful. The reality is better than the image, for those who talk about their experiences are usually those who have been disturbed and their reaction is as much due to the sensitivity of the issue as to the insensitivity of the official. No matter how kind and understanding he may be some old people are so tense that they perceive suspicion in an innocent pause and see sarcasm in a reassuring smile.

Elderly people should be encouraged to apply for supplementary pension if they are having financial difficulties. If they are considered eligible they not only receive the basic amount necessary for food, fuel, and other necessities. They will receive their rent and rates and the interest on any outstanding mortgage which has still to be paid. They are also eligible for help with other expenses, notably heating costs (see p. 182) and for the cost of fares to visit relatives in hospital, and they may be able to claim a lump sum for replacement of expensive items of clothing or household effects.

The over-80s pension

This pension, sometimes called 'the old person's pension', is paid to very elderly people who were unable to make sufficient national insurance contributions which were only started in 1948. People aged over 80 who are in financial difficulty should apply, using leaflet NI 184. No means test is required for the granting of this pension.

Help with health charges

Elderly people are eligible for free prescriptions, glasses, and dental treatment whether or not they qualify for retirement or widow's pensions and irrespective of their income or wealth (leaflet M11 – free dental treatment, free glasses, free prescriptions, free milk and vitamins – gives full details of these benefits).

War pensions

Pensions are paid to people who were disabled in War, either as a serviceman, merchant seaman, or civilian. The amount paid varies depending on the degree of disability and on the rank of the recipient. Widows, widowers, and orphans of people who die as a result of service in the forces may also be eligible for a pension. If an old person is receiving a war pension the general practitioner need not worry unduly about their financial problems because the war pensions branch of Social Security has welfare officers who keep in touch with war pensioners. They ensure that the old person is receiving all the statutory benefits for which he is eligible and they can tap charitable regimental funds for small lump sums such as £50 to help in a crisis. The war pensions welfare officer can be contacted via the local social security office or by writing to the Controller, War Pensions, DHSS, Norcross, Blackpool, FY5 3TA.

Benefits for disabled people

In the nineteen-sixties it was appreciated that some disabled people were treated unjustly. Those who had been disabled as a result of war or of the effects of an industrial disease received more social security than those whose disabilities could not be attributed to those causes. Furthermore, those whose disabilities developed at an early age and who were prevented from working and therefore from paying National Insurance contributions were much worse off than those who became disabled later in life and who had therefore been able to pay sufficient contributions to qualify for National Insurance benefits. To help disadvantaged disabled people two very important benefits were introduced – the Attendance Allowance and the Invalid Care Allowance.

Attendance allowance

This is paid to people suffering from physical or mental disability who require frequent attention either with self-care or for their own safety or the safety of others. The person must have needed the help for six months before the claim is made. The allowance is paid at two rates: at a higher rate – £23.65 in 1980 – if attendance is required both day and night, and at a lower rate – £15.75 in 1981 – if help is required either by day or by night. If a person receiving the lower rate deteriorates the allowance can be increased to the higher rate.

The person's general practitioner is not required to write a report. All that is required is for the disabled person to complete, or for someone else to complete, the claim form in leaflet NI 205 but a letter of support from the general practitioner can alert the doctor who visit from the Attendance Allowance Board to aspects of the disabled person's dependence which may not be immediately obvious. However, a letter of support is very useful when application is being made for a lower allowance to be increased to the higher rate.

The Attendance Allowance is normally paid in addition to supplementary pension and all other social security benefits, except the constant attendance allowance which some war pensioners receive, and is tax free.

Invalid care allowance

The Attendance Allowance is very useful and can meet the costs of extra heating required by a disabled person or the cost of new clothes and bed clothes or to pay someone to help the old person. It therefore reduces the elder's economic dependence on her relatives and relieves the financial burden on them. The invalid care allowance was introduced to help relatives who not only had to support a disabled old person but who were unable to work because of their commitment. It is paid to men and single women of working age who are unable to work because they have to stay at home to look after a severely disabled relative, that is one who is receiving an Attendance Allowance. Application is made by using the form in leaflet NI 212. A doctor's letter is not usually necessary unless the claim is turned down and the relative wishes to appeal against the decision.

Because the Invalid Care Allowance is only about half the amount recognized by the Department of Health and Social Security as necessary for subsistence the recipient should also apply to the Social Security office for a supplementary allowance and may be eligible for other benefits, for example free glasses, free prescriptions, and free dental treatment. The person in receipt of an invalid care allowance automatically receives one very important benefit – Class I National Insurance contribution. This is credited to her so that she becomes eligible for sickness or unemployment benefit and for a retirement pension when she reaches pension age just as she would if she were in paid employment.

Sources of advice

The general practitioner can obtain advice about social security from the health visitor, the social services department, the Citizens' Advice Bureau, or the local office of Age Concern. In addition he can consult the concise and clear leaflet 'Which Benefit? 60 Ways to Get Cash Help' (DHSS leaflet FB2) or 'Your Rights', Age Concern's excellent booklet.

In addition to these two booklets the health centre or surgery should have copies of the following leaflets:

NP 32	Your retirement pension.
NI 205	Attendance Allowance.
NI 212	Invalid Care Allowance.
NI 184	Non-contributory retirement pension for people over 80.
NP 32A	Your retirement pension if widowed or divorced.
SB1	Cash help from supplementary benefit.
H11	Your hosptial fares.
M11	Free milk and vitamins, glasses, dental treatment, and prescriptions.
NI 149	Death grant.

If it proves difficult to obtain these from a local post office they can be obtained from DHSS (Leaflets), PO Box 21, Stanmore, Middlesex, HA7 1AY. When ordering leaflets, and the Leaflets Office will send whatever number of each is required, it is wise to ask for a copy of leaflet NI 146 – 'Catalogue of Social Security Leaflets' which lists all the leaflets available and includes an order form.

PROBLEMS WITH PRIVATE INCOME

Not all older people depend on Social Security. Many have private incomes either from employment or occupational pensions or from investment. Such people may also have problems, as capital diminishes or shares fall on the market or as inflation diminishes the value of their pension. This type of financial problem can be very difficult to manage because the person affected may try to keep up appearances and conceal her difficulties until a crisis occurs.

If the person has capital, even if the only capital is their house, a solution can often be found, for example by the purchase of an annuity, but the options are difficult to evaluate without advice. The bank manager is the best source of advice in the first instance and elderly people will receive sound advice from bank managers even though their assets are small. If the person does not have a bank account she should be encouraged to open one either with one of the major clearing banks or with the Trustee Savings Bank who give excellent advice to people with low incomes and small amounts of capital.

There is a new Age Concern publication called 'Your Taxes' which is very useful for elderly people who have a private income.

HOUSING PROBLEMS

Effects

Elderly people live in worse housing conditions than young people. The dwellings they inhabit are, in general, older and they less frequently have all the basic amenities – hot water, an inside toilet, and a bathroom – than those of younger people. Paradoxically, older people state that they are, on average, more statisfied with their housing than younger people, even though it lacks amenities or central heating more frequently, and the reasons for this have been discussed previously (see p. 116). However, many old people are dissatisfied with their housing conditions and bad housing can cause or aggravate the following problems:

1. Depression; remember also that depression may be the cause of the person's housing problem for it may be the reason why she is neglecting her property.
2. Anxiety.
3. Hypothermia (see p. 45).
4. Incontinence (see p. 50).
5. Institutionalization; the provision of domiciliary support is much more difficult if the housing conditions are poor. It is, for example, difficult to provide an adequate nursing service for a very dependent old person if the nurse has to heat water in a bucket on the gas stove before she can give her a bath. Similarly, support at home is much more difficult to organize if the old person requires to have a coal fire lit seven days a week and if she has to use a commode because she can no longer reach an outside toilet.

Elderly patients often say 'I want to move' but a move is not always the best solution to their problem (Fig. 10.3).

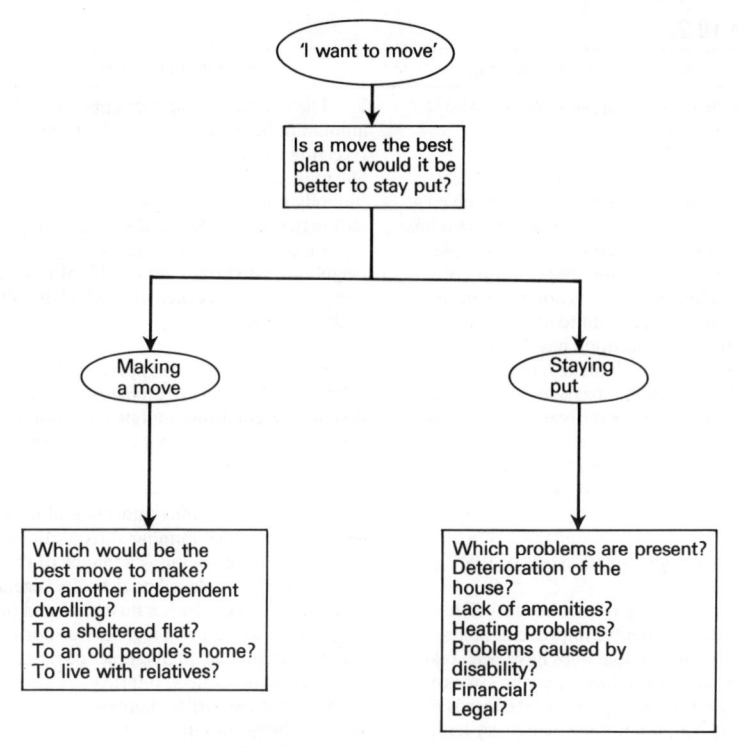

```
                    ┌─────────────────┐
                    │  'I want to move'│
                    └────────┬────────┘
                             ▼
                    ┌─────────────────┐
                    │ Is a move the best│
                    │ plan or would it be│
                    │ better to stay put?│
                    └────────┬────────┘
                   ┌─────────┴─────────┐
                   ▼                   ▼
              ┌─────────┐         ┌─────────┐
              │ Making  │         │ Staying │
              │ a move  │         │  put    │
              └────┬────┘         └────┬────┘
```

┌──────────────────────────┐   ┌──────────────────────────┐
│ Which would be the   │   │ Which problems are present?│
│ best move to make?   │   │ Deterioration of the   │
│ To another independent   │   │ house?   │
│ dwelling?   │   │ Lack of amenities?   │
│ To a sheltered flat?   │   │ Heating problems?   │
│ To an old people's home? │   │ Problems caused by   │
│ To live with relatives? │   │ disability?   │
└──────────────────────────┘   │ Financial?   │
                                  │ Legal?   │
                                  └──────────────────────────┘

Fig. 10.3. Housing choices.

Staying put or making a move

Even when good reasons for moving house can be identified the benefits of staying put and the difficulties which may result from moving, particularly the difficulty in making friends if one is immobile and house-bound, must always be taken into account and should not be underestimated (Table 10.2).

In general the old person should be encouraged to stay put unless there is a very good reason for making a move. She should be helped to think of all the advantages and disadvantages of moving and of remaining in her own dwelling and given time to make a careful decision. She should also be helped to explore what is possible for the decision to remain where she is may be made for her, if, for example, she is told that she may have to wait five or more years even if she decided that she wished to be rehoused. The first step in helping an old person with a housing problem is to see if it is possible for her to stay put.

Staying put

There are five common types of problem which interfere with an old person's ability to stay in her own dwelling (Table 10.3):

184 *Social problems*

Table 10.2.

Good reasons for moving	Disadvantages of moving
1. To be nearer a daughter or son who is willing to help	1. The old person may not appreciate the amount of help and support which she is receiving from the community in which she lives. She may say that 'no-one comes to see me', or 'nobody is interested in me round here', although this may not be the case because the old person omits to mention, or forgets, the neighbour who brings her in a bit of baking every week or the corner shop which is willing to deliver groceries
2. To move away from an environment which was once liked but is now perceived as an alien or threatening culture because it has 'gone down', or because coloured people have bought a large number of properties. A fear of coloured people is not uncommon and can be very difficult to assuage. Even when the neighbourhood has developed characteristics which make it easy to understand the old person's aversion it is important not to underestimate the contribution which the community is making; not infrequently the neighbours of whom the elder is afraid are willing to help and are keeping an eye on her	2. She may also fail to appreciate that neighbours keep an eye on her and would be prepared to challenge anyone who looked suspicious whom they saw in her garden or at her door
3. To overcome isolation (see p. 195)	3. The old person may underestimate the contribution which familiar surroundings make to her mental well-being. The shape of the hall in which her sons played cricket; the vegetable patch once worked by her husband; and the bedroom in which her daughter was born are poignant reminders of a happier past and may be the cause of sadness, but they are also full of memories of the earlier chapters of the old person's biography and are therefore important to her self-consciousness
4. To move away from a house which is impossible to repair or improve or adapt. Even after all possible steps have been taken to improve the dwelling it may be impossible to make it suitable by normal standards but some old people continue living very happily in dwellings which are 'unfit'	

Table 10.3.

Type of problem	Typical problem	Solution: advice for old people and their relatives
Deterioration or dilapidation	Minor problems such as leaking taps or a broken window pane. Major problems such as faulty wiring or a leaking roof	Grants and loans are available, ask the advice of the environmental health officer
Lack of amenities	Lack of inside toilet or bath or hot water	Grants and loans are available, ask the advice of the environmental health officer
Problems caused by the onset of disability	Inability to reach upstairs toilet or bathroom	Ask the advice of the domiciliary occupational therapist
Financial problems	Difficulty with rates and rent	Claim rate or rent rebate
Legal problems	Threat of eviction	Seek the advice of the Citizens' Advice Bureau or Housing Aid Centre

Deterioration and dilapidation.
Lack of amenities.
Problems caused by the onset of disability.
Financial problems (Table 10.4).
Legal problems.

Usually an officer from the Town Hall will be available to visit housebound people to explain the system of help with rent and rates and to help them apply.

The environmental health officer merits special mention. Until 1974 the public health inspector was managed by the medical officer of health but was granted his independence in 1974 on the reorganization of local government, changing his title to environmental health officer in the process. The EHO has a

Table 10.4. *Financial help with housing costs*

Type of tenure	Benefits available	Where to apply
Owner-occupier	Rate rebates	Town Hall or Council Offices
Council tenant	Rate rebate Rent rebate	Housing Department
Private tenant	Rate rebate Rent allowance	Town Hall or Council Offices

wide range of responsibilities, such as health and safety at work, the investigation of food poisoning, and the inspection and supervision of shops and restaurants. However, one major part of his work concerns housing problems and the list which follows covers some of the more common types of problem with which the EHO deals:

- Problems of owner-occupiers, such as dampness, condensation, structural damage, lack of amenities, blocked drains, and dry rot. To solve these problems the environmental health officer can help the old person to apply for house renovation grants and council loans which cover the cost of the work not covered by the grant.
- Problems with landlords, such as an unwillingness to repair or improve the dwelling. Environmental health officers have many powers to deal with this type of problem but are well aware of the fear which the tenant has of the landlord's power so are very diplomatic in their approach.
- Problems with neighbours such as noise or smells.
- Problems with rats, mice, cockroaches, and other pests.

Most environmental health officers are accustomed to, and are skilled at, speaking to elderly people and a referral can be made to the environmental health department with as much confidence that the elder will be sympathetically treated as can a referral to any other professional service. Environmental health officers are not used often enough by doctors or other professionals in the health and social services.

Making a move

There are four main options:
1. Moving to live with relatives.
2. Another more suitable dwelling.
3. A sheltered flat.
4. An old people's home.

To relatives

In general this is undesirable. If it is possible it is better to live with relatives rather than near them (see p. 145).

To sheltered housing or a non-sheltered dwelling

Sheltered housing is often considered to be the ideal solution for an old person with housing problems but its contribution is more limited than is sometimes appreciated. The warden is employed to keep an eye on the tenants in the scheme, usually by calling once a day, and to mobilize the appropriate health and social services should problems develop. She is not employed to prepare meals, to do shopping or housework, to administer medication, or to perform simple nursing tasks. Sheltered housing is, therefore, not necessarily the solution to the problem of a person who is very disabled or confused. In fact it can be a great mistake to rehouse confused elderly people in sheltered housing because they may annoy the other tenants, with whom they live in such close proximity, and be further confused by the warden's visits and surveillance.

Because the warden is usually single-handed and lives in the scheme seven days a week she is in a very difficult position. Even though she, and the tenants and their relatives, are told that she is officially off-duty at certain times the personal characteristics which made her apply for the job of warden may make it impossible for her to be emotionally off-duty and she may worry continually about tenants whom she feels are not eating properly or who are at risk. This may develop until she herself becomes exhausted or depressed or the consequence may be that she develops an aggressive approach to the doctor whom she sees as the person who is responsible for the continuing residence of an old person whom the warden believes should be in a hospital or old people's home.

For elderly people who are very isolated or who are very nervous of being alone, perhaps as a consequence of a break-in, sheltered housing may be the best option although it is often possible to provide sufficient support and reassurance without moving them by overcoming their isolation (see p. 195) or by the provision of a phone (see p. 173). For other elderly people a move to an ordinary flat will usually be adequate if it proves impossible to improve or adapt the dwelling in which they are living.

How to move house

Elderly council tenants can move house with relative ease. The local authority is usually keen to rehouse them in a small dwelling because it will gain a three-bedroomed house if it helps them move, but a letter from the old person's general practitioner to the housing department or, if confidential information is relevant, to the community physician is often helpful.

Elderly owner-occupiers can, in theory, sell their house and buy a smaller more suitable dwelling but in practice the capital realized by the sale of a deteriorating house is often insufficient to buy a modern flat or bungalow. Many owner-occupiers must therefore apply to the local authority or to a housing association for rehousing, as private tenants have to do. Housing associations are funded by central government and are not run by local authorities, although both build identical dwellings, which means that they do not require the same residence qualifications as local authorities; that is they are prepared to accept applications and to rehouse elderly people who do not live locally and they are therefore particularly useful for the old person who wishes to move from one part of the country to another. The local authority housing department will supply a list of the housing associations which have flats for elderly people within its boundaries. A letter of support from the general practitioner is always useful when elderly owner-occupiers or private tenants are applying for rehousing but the doctor is not always able to claim a fee from the health or local authority, except when he has been specifically asked to provide a medical report.

To an old people's home

Old people's homes have been criticized but for some old people who are tired of struggling at home, nervous and isolated residential care is the best option.

The need of an individual for residential care is determined by five factors:
1. Physical disability.
2. Availability of community services.
3. Personality.
4. Mental state.
5. Attitudes of other people.

Community services: the level of physical disability is obviously important but it is influenced by the other factors. The length of time which a disabled dependent person is able to continue living in his own home is also a function of the amount of help which she is able to receive from community health and social services. She will be able to live at home much longer if she can be given home help and domiciliary nursing seven days a week than if there are only sufficient resources for her to be given help four days a week. In our opinion no old person should have to go to live in a home until life at home with at least one visit from a home help and two from a district nurse seven days a week has been tried.

Personality: some of the elderly people who are admitted to homes are less disabled than others who carry on living at home either because their motivation is weaker or because they are less rewarding. The person's biography is very helpful for the person who is poorly motivated in old age was usually of the same nature when younger. If she was not, a reason for the

188 Social problems

change in personality, commonly depression, should be sought. Similarly, not all old people are equally rewarding and an elderly person who is self-centred or who is ungrateful and critical of the help given her will be supported by relatives, friends, and neighbours for a shorter period of time than the cheerful person who is interested in, and concerned for, the problems of other people and who minimizes her own difficulties.

Mental state: an old person who is very confused may be unable to manage at home even though she is not severely physically disabled. Unfortunately such people are often unacceptable to the staff of an old people's home.

Attitudes of others: often the demands for home admission come from exhausted relatives (see p. 140).

Residential care checklist

Before deciding that a move to residential care alternatives should be reviewed:
  1. What does the old person want?
  2. Could the old person's level of disability be reduced? (see pp. 107, 156).
  3. Could the domiciliary occupational therapist do anything more to help her to become more independent?
  4. Could she be given more help at home?
  5. Would day care relieve her or her supporters?
  6. Would a planned series of short-stay admissions help her or her supporters?

How to move to a home

There are three types of old people's home – local authority, voluntary, and private. Application for a place in a local authority home is made to the Social Services Department or, in Scotland, the Social Work Department.

The social services department can provide a list of the private and voluntary homes in the area but may be unable or unwilling to give a critical appraisal of the suitability of a home to an old person or her relatives. GRACE (Mrs Gould's Residential Advisory Centre for the Elderly), Leigh Corner, Leigh Hill Road, Cobham, Surrey, is an excellent source of advice about homes in the south of England, and the Counsel and Care for the Elderly (see p. 111) is also able to give advice on homes. The supervision of private nursing homes for old people is the responsibility of the health service and the community physician will be able to provide a list of the nursing homes in the district. In practice there is little difference between nursing homes for old people and private or voluntary old people's homes.

Those who move to a local authority home are 'means tested' and have to pay according to their means, which is a cause of great betterness to those who have struggled to save or buy a house or earn an occupational pension. Those who go to live in private or voluntary homes can apply for the Attendance Allowance and supplementary benefit and the health authority or social services department may be able to make a contribution if the person's income is insufficient to meet the cost.

Problems with moving

The move to the home can have a deleterious effect on the old person's physical and mental condition which is known as the negative relocation effect. This can be minimized if the old person is given time to adapt to the new home and the social worker will try to facilitate this by arranging day care and short stays at the home before the definitive move is made. The general practitioner can also help by keeping in close touch with the old person at this time and by keeping her on his list for the first few months after the move.

Too fit but too frail

An increasingly common problem for general practitioners is the person who is too fit for hospital but too frail for an old people's home. Sometimes all three types of institution become involved and the general practitioner is left supporting an old person who is not considered confused enough for a long-term psychiatric bed nor sufficiently disabled for a long-term geriatric bed, but who is not considered fit enough for an old people's home, even though everyone agrees that she should be 'in somewhere' (Fig. 10.4; Table 10.5). This type of problem can be frustrating and time consuming.

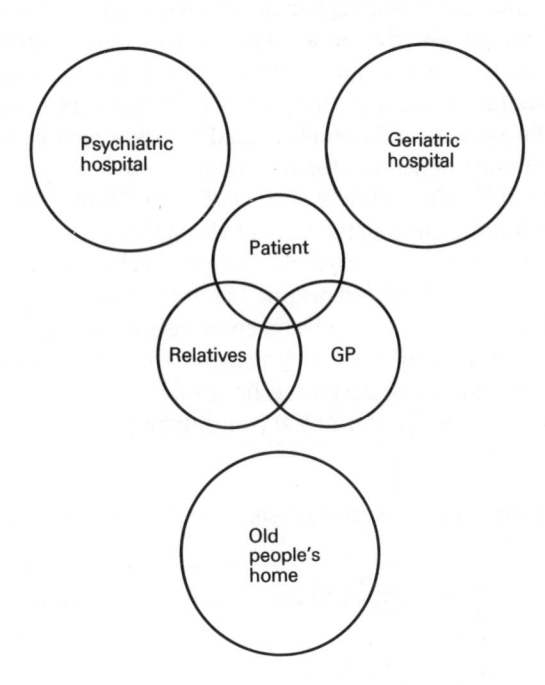

Fig. 10.4. Too fit but too frail.

190   *Social problems*

Table 10.5. *Possible approaches to the 'too fit–too frail' problem*

Possible approaches	Limitations
1. Increase domiciliary support	May be unavailable. Of little use to old people living with families
2. Increase day care or use short-stay admissions	May be unavailable. Can aggravate confusion. Old person may refuse.
3. Try to find a private home	Financial costs of private care
4. Ask for case conference	May be waste of time but may bring both, or all three, sides together productively
5. Refer to District Medical Officer	May not achieve solution but will keep him informed of type of problem causing difficulty for general practitioners

HEATING PROBLEMS (see p. 45)

Some elderly people are particularly at risk of hypothermia because of certain physiological and pathological changes but very few would develop hypothermia if they lived in a well heated environment; physical factors predispose to hypothermia, social factors precipitate the condition. Hypothermia is not the only problem; cold and fear of heating bills are common causes of suffering. Furthermore the old person who lives in a cold environment is a source of anxiety to her friends, relatives, neighbours in winter and they make many calls on the general practitioner to 'do something', which often means to persuade the old person to go into a home. Old people in cold houses generate unnecessary work for the general practitioner and for the district nurse and home help who have to work in very difficult conditions (Fox *et al.* 1973) (Table 10.6).

The proportion who say that they are cold is small but this reflects the hardness of the generation because a much higher proportion have no form of heating in rooms in which we would regard heating as normal (Table 10.7).

There are three steps which can be taken to ensure a warmer dwelling:

1. Increasing the amount of money available for heating costs.
2. Burning that money in the most efficient way.
3. Reducing the amount of heat lost by insulating the old person, bed, room, and house.

Table 10.6. *Percentage of elderly people who are not warm enough in certain rooms*

	Men	Women
In bed	7.4	7.6
In living room	8.8	8.2
In kitchen	11.6	12.2

From Hunt, A. (1978). *The elderly at home*, p. 80. HMSO, London.

Table 10.7. *Percentage of elderly households with no heating in certain rooms*

Room	Percentage without heating
Bedroom	29.7
Hall and passage	51.7
Bathroom	37.7
Lavatory	60.0
Kitchen	48.9

From Hunt, A. (1978). *The elderly at home*, p. 48–50. HMSO, London.

Meeting heating costs

Heating costs constitute a significant part of the total budget of an old person and the first steps should be to encourage her and her supporters to review the whole of her income and to ensure that she is claiming all the benefits for which she is eligible (see p. 181). In addition an elderly person who receives a supplementary pension ('social security' – see p. 177) may be eligible for an extra allowance to help with heating costs if she has to use central heating with a fixed cost or if she lives in a dwelling which is difficult to heat or if she suffers from a disease which increases her need for warmth such as an immobilizing disease or one which puts her at greater than average risk of hypothermia. A letter from the general practitioner is very useful in such cases and it should be given to the old person or to the person who is applying on her behalf. If the old person who is having difficulty with heating costs is not receiving supplementary pension she can write to the social security office and ask if she is in fact eligible for a supplementary pension, and thus for a heating allowance, because many eligible older people are not receiving a supplementary pension.

Poverty is a cause of heating problems which is often difficult to solve but an even greater difficulty is presented by the old person who had sufficient money but who refuses to spend it on heating; sometimes the person has a very great deal of money but refuses to spend it. One reason for this is that the old person has always been used to a cold dwelling and does not see why she should live in a warmer environment just because she is old. The old person may be persuaded to use more heat if her general practitioner explains why she is at greater risk of hypothermia than she was when she was younger.

A more common reason is fear of debt – 'there's one thing, doctor; if I were to drop down dead I wouldn't owe a penny to anyone'. Fear of debt is linked to the fear of the Workhouse which still haunts some old people, because the Workhouse was the place to which impoverished old people were admitted. Not only do they fear debt but many older people feel that they are no longer able to control their expenditure as they once could and this can be very frightening. They were accustomed to buy coal, which they could see before they used it, and they were able to budget their coal by watching the level in the bunker fall or by watching the heap in the cellar diminish. Now they are expected to use an invisible commodity which is measured in incomprehensible units –

192 *Social problems*

Watts or BTUs – before they pay for it and are unused to the concept of quarterly bills which may be much bigger than their weekly income.

To overcome such difficulties is not easy and it may prove to be impossible. It may help if the general practitioner emphasizes the need for warmth, giving 'doctor's orders' if necessary (see p. 177), but it is equally important to help the old person with her budgeting by ensuring that someone helps her purchase pre-payment fuel stamps every week, and repeatedly reassures her that she need not fear disconnection, eviction or condemnation if she does get into debt.

Burning money efficiently

Not only do old people have less money to spend on heating they also burn their money much less efficiently than younger people because they use inefficient heating apparatus in poor repair. For example, the radiant electric fire is a very inefficient source of heat but it is used very often by older people.

Sources of financial help

Financial help may be available from social services or social security to meet the costs of replacing an inefficient heat source or one which is in dangerously poor repair but, as is often the case, it may be difficult to raise the small amount which it is necessary to spend to reduce the running costs of a household with a low income. Remember that the old person's former employer, or his former regiment, or the regiment in which a deceased spouse served, are often willing to give a lump sum to help.

If the old person cannot use her source of heating because of disability, for example because she is too disabled by arthritis to make up a coal fire, the domiciliary occupational therapist may be able to arrange for a replacement paid for under the Chronically Sick and Disabled Persons Act.

Problems with central heating

Those people who have central heating face different types of problems, and often very large bills. Some people are unable to control the system efficiently, either because they cannot reach, or read, or manipulate or understand the thermostat and the time clock. They therefore use the system very inefficiently, for example by leaving it on all the time and opening all the windows, or they switch it off completely and use paraffin or radiant electric heaters. To help such people it is best to ask the gas or electricity office to send a domestic adviser to instruct the old person and, if possible, her supporters how best to set the thermostat and time clock.

Reducing heat loss

It is essential to help the old person minimize heat loss by more effective insulation.

Warm food

Unnecessary heat loss can be prevented if warm food or drink is consumed rather than cold food or drink. If the old person is unable to manage to cook for herself and is alone for long periods of time it should be suggested to her supporters that a thermos flask, or better, two or three flasks, should be introduced to her daily routine so that she always has warm drinks such as tea, milk, cocoa, and soup, to hand.

Warm clothes

The elder's ability to dress must be reviewed (see p. 164) but it is also necessary to ask whether the old person has sufficient warm clothes to put on. If she has not the domiciliary occupational therapist should be able to help choose suitable warm clothes, if she has been involved because the old person had to be taught how to dress. If the domiciliary occupational therapist has not been involved the home help or a relative or friend can help if an occupational therapist is not involved. Mail order catalogues are a useful means of shopping but a visit to the shops, with the help of voluntary transport (see p. 169) is even better.

Fewer draughts

Voluntary helpers can be enlisted to do these jobs, they can insulate windows and doors to reduce draughts, but remember that the most effective way of reducing draughts round the door is to warm the rest of the house; a warm room and a freezing hall is a recipe for draughts no matter how well the door has been insulated.

More insulation

It is often possible to insulate the room in which the old person sits by lining curtains, or by blocking off an unused fireplace, provided that paraffin or bottled gas heaters are not being used for they can be dangerous if there is insufficient ventilation. Loft insulation is also important and grants are available from the environmental health department to help with the cost.

Warmth in the bedroom

The elderly person may need encouragement not to sleep with her window open on cold nights and she should also be advised to heat her bedroom, if only for thirty minutes before retiring to bed, even though she has never done so before. The bedclothes may be thin and need replacing. The old person should be encouraged to try a continental quilt and it is also worth while suggesting that she try a low voltage electric blanket. A number of different models have been developed for the use of elderly people being cheap to run and safe. Some can even be left on all night and are safe when wet by incontinence. The purchase of these blankets for donation to the district nursing service to lend to old people is an excellent focus for voluntary fund-raising efforts and the idea should be suggested to local groups. If the old person does not want an electric blanket it should be ensured that she can fill a hot water bottle safely.

Warmth checklist

1. Has she as much money as possible?
2. Is she willing to spend it?
3. Is she spending her money as efficiently as she could?
4. Could she have more warm food and drink?
5. Could she be more warmly dressed?
6. Could her room be better insulated and have fewer draughts?
7. Could she be warmer in bed?
8. Could her whole house be better insulated?

Fire risks

Even greater than the anxiety felt by relatives, neighbours, and friends about hypothermia is the anxiety felt about fire and considerable pressure may be exerted on the doctor to persuade the old person to enter a home 'for her own safety'. The increased risk is real and the mortality from fire increases sharply in older age groups, although there is no evidence that other people are often harmed. Almost always the only sufferer is the old person. When a person has been referred as 'a fire risk' two steps are appropriate: firstly the identification of specific dangers and secondly prompt action.

Heating apparatus is a common cause of anxiety, especially paraffin heaters, but they are not dangerous provided that they are properly serviced and maintained. Old paraffin heaters in poor repair can constitute a risk and the elder should be encouraged to use another form of heating. Coal fires should be safely guarded if the old person is unsteady on her feet and gas fires should have an automatic lighting device. If a new gas fire is being installed one should be chosen which has controls on top where they are easily accessible and not on the bottom.

Cookers are another cause for concern but the smell of a burning pan usually alerts neighbours or the old person herself before a serious fire starts. The old person who leaves an unlit gas ring is a cause of serious anxiety to those concerned for her and for her neighbours but this problem can be solved if a gas cooker with an automatic pilot light is installed.

The most common causes of fires in old age are cigarettes and matches and although an old person should be advised not to smoke in bed old habits are hard to change. A more feasible approach is to try to replace the matches with a lighter but even this simple suggestion may be rejected.

Whatever is decided to be done it should be done promptly because the anxiety of other people can be reduced, even if the risk of fire is not markedly reduced, provided that they feel that their anxiety is being taken seriously and that something is being done. If, for example, relatives are advised to arrange a gas safety check and to give the old person a lighter their anxiety may be reduced to tolerable levels even though the risk of fire is not significantly reduced. If the anxiety of the old person's supporters can be reduced they will often be willing to continue helping her whereas they were putting pressure on her to go into a home because they found the anxiety intolerable.

The management of fire risks should focus just as much on the management of the anxieties of other people as on the reduction of the risk. As is so often the case the anxieties of other people are among the most important factors which the doctor has to manage to help the old person to live on at home.

ISOLATION

Isolation is a difficult problem to detect or even discuss because there are no objective criteria such as temperature or haemoglobin concentration against which the old person's condition can be assessed. The number of people whom the old person meets each week is obviously important but the quality of each meeting is also important. A half hour's discussion with a loved daughter is obviously more rewarding than a friendly wave from the postman; the former may be called a social engagement whereas the latter is a social contact and it is the number of social engagements which is the more helpful indicator.

Nevertheless it is insufficient merely to try to count the number of social engagements because the effect of the isolation to the old person is influenced by other factors. The old person who was 'never much of a one for going out' and 'always enjoyed my own company' will probably be less disturbed by isolation than the person who has always been gregarious so the biography of the individual is always important. Nevertheless some people are able to adapt to isolation better than others but adaptability is not an easy quality to measure either. It is not related solely to educational status, although the old person who does enjoy reading and has always has a number of interests which do not require the company of others will usually adapt more easily. In the absence of any definite criteria it is therefore necessary to look for the effects of isolation if it appears that the person has become isolated, rather than to spend much time trying to determine how isolated he or she is in comparison with other people.

Effects

There are four common effects:
    loneliness;
    mental disorders;
    nutritional problems;
    dependence.

Loneliness

Not all isolated people are lonely, and some lonely old people are not isolated, but loneliness should always be considered when a person has become isolated even though he does not complain that he is lonely, or even denies it when asked. It may be that the elder does not wish to admit his loneliness to others as part of his strategy for coping with his loneliness, as old people often adopt the 'I'm all right' approach when they are coping with a problem which they believe to be insoluble (see p. 117). Another reason for a denial of loneliness may be that the old person is afraid that if he admits he is lonely the response of others will be to say that 'you should go and live in an old people's home where there are nice lounges with lots of people to talk to'.

Mental disorder

Depression is an obvious consequence of loneliness but isolation can cause other types of mental disorder. Disorientation in time and space, apathy, and paranoid thoughts have all been shown to result from isolation and in research on 'brainwashing' it has been demonstrated that these symptoms can be produced within forty-eight hours in young fit soldiers. Many older people are alone for seventy hours every weekend from Friday morning, when the home help leaves, to Monday morning when she returns. Not only are old people isolated; they are often less able to divert their attention because of visual and hearing impairment. To describe the mental consequence of isolation as being either affective, or intellectual, or motivational is inadequate; the isolated person's whole personality can waste away. Man is a social being and a person who is isolated and who is not interacting with other people may start to show changes in all aspects of his personality which are similar to those produced by dementia. Dementia is a cause of isolation and people who suffer from dementia are more severely affected by isolation but, unfortunately, the contribution of isolation to their mental deterioration is often overlooked, because it is assumed that every mental symptom is due to dementia.

Nutritional problems

Nutritional problems are more likely among isolated people because eating is, for most people, a social activity with the meal as a meeting. In some people the physiological hunger drives are insufficiently strong to overcome the loss of appetite which may result from isolation. Visits to a lunch club are, in general, more effective than meals on wheels although they are more difficult to arrange. They are more effective because some people who receive meals on wheels do not eat them because they are, necessarily, left to eat them alone. To complicate the assessment even further it is often very difficult to assess how much of the meal is actually eaten because the old person may not wish to reveal that she is not eating the meals because she has become dependent on the visits of the person delivering the meals on wheels to alleviate her isolation, as she may become dependent on any other service.

Dependence

Many isolated old people become dependent on the professionals who may constitute the major part of their social life. The relationships which commence on professional terms become personal relationships, as it is right that they should. However, this has its disadvantages and one of the principal drawbacks is that a person who is dependent on professionals for her social wellbeing has little incentive to become less disabled because a reduction in her disability will result in an increase in her isolation.

A young man who has fractured his shaft of femur has every incentive to co-operate with professionals; he does so in the expectation that he will be back on the saddle of his Yamaha within six months. However, the old person who suffers from a number of chronic disabling diseases is in a different position. In many cases he will not get back to a full social life if he complies with medical treatment and the advice of the occupational and physiotherapists. The old person appreciates, usually unconsciously, that if she takes the drugs which have been prescribed and does everything that the physiotherapist says and uses the board and seat provided by the domiciliary occupational therapist so that she can bath herself, the consequence will be that the district nurse will no longer come. Similarly, if she works as hard as she can and regains her independence to manage in the kitchen her 'reward' will be that the home help's visits will be reduced.

Mrs. T. was 82 and immobilized by osteoarthritis and she also had a large varicose ulcer. She had very few visitors but the nurse called three times a week to dress her ulcer. Her only trip out of her house was on the alternate weekends which she spent in the dermatology ward for ulcer treatment. Although neither depressed nor demented she would not put her leg up and never went to bed. At first she said it was because of the stairs but when the bed was brought down to the room in which she sat she still refused to go to bed saying that she was 'all right' in the chair. The main obstacle to compliance in her case was that her ulcer ensured that she had a social life.

Therefore neither 'healing', nor 'cure', nor 'independence' may be sufficiently attractive objectives to ensure good compliance if the old person knows or fears that the attainment of the objective will result in a greater degree of isolation.

Causes

A decade ago the 'disengagement theory' was popular. It argued that old people naturally withdrew from society as they grew older, like snails withdrawing into their shells, but this theory is no longer accepted. It is uncommon for someone to become isolated voluntarily; there is usually some reason over which they have no control but the person's personality is, however, relevant. Elderly people who are unrewarding to visit – those who are bitter and self-centered or those who criticize everything that is done for them and never show any gratitude – are much more likely to become isolated if they become housebound by disability than the person who is uncomplaining, interested in the problems of other people, and grateful for what is done for her. If it is thought that the person is isolated because the visit is unrewarding it is important to consider her biography, to try to determine whether her bitter, critical and self-centred attitude has always been her approach to life or whether it is a new feature. If it is the latter it may be a reaction to isolation and disability or a symptom of depression. In most cases the person's personality is not the principal cause of her isolation.

There are six causes of isolation which are much more common. Each may be complicated by poverty because many old people are unable to use public transport but cannot afford to run a car or hire taxis.

1. Immobility (see p. 45).
2. Instability – falling or fear of falling (see p. 31).
3. Incontinence or fear of incontinence (see p. 48).
4. Sensory deprivation (see p. 35).
5. Dementia.
6. The death of friends.

Treatment and alleviation

The first line of treatment is obviously the treatment of the underlying cause but it is often impossible to cure it completely so efforts must be directed to the alleviation of isolation. This can be done in three ways:

1. By trying to arrange for more people to visit the old person at home, which can be difficult because volunteers are often unwilling to take on the long-term commitment of regular visiting, often because they are afraid that the old person will become emotionally dependent on them.

2. It is important to try to provide more stimulation in her home when the old person is alone. The means of doing this are by trying to ensure that the old person has a clock and a calendar; by trying to ensure that she has a working radio and television; by encouraging the old person to read more and to use the volunteer book delivery service run by most libraries; and by helping the elder to consider benefits that a pet might confer. The ownership of a pet has several benefits other than the company the pet offers, the most important of which is the fact that the pet is dependent on the old person and this is very valuable.

3. Every attempt should be made to arrange for the old person to go out more, often to re-establish the broken links with the church or club or pub. This can be much more difficult than it appears and the old person may be very resistant to the idea of going out. This may be due to the fact that she is ashamed of her appearance or her clothes, or because she is afraid that she will be incontinent, or because she has lost or fears that she has lot, her social skills. It is, therefore, sometimes necessary to encourage the person to have her hair done at home and to buy new clothes, and to ask friends or volunteers to help her with these preparations. It may be necessary to emphasize that she will not be incontinent or to provide the means by which incontinence can be concealed, for example by the provision of Kanga pants. Occasionally an old person is so reluctant to leave her home even after the practical problems have been solved that she may be considered to be agoraphobic and in such cases the advice of a clinical psychologist or psychiatrist is indicated.

11 Practical issues facing the general practitioner in caring for the elderly

Peter Pritchard

INTRODUCTION

This chapter is in three sections. In the first, I will discuss whether we as general practitioners face serious problems in coping with our elderly patients now and in the future.

In the second section I will consider preventive measures which a general practitioner and staff might undertake in order to keep the problem under control. In particular, attention will be focused on prevention of arterial disease; on the early diagnosis and treatment of disabling conditions; and on prevention of accidents.

The third section is about measures which can be undertaken now to help us deal with the current situation. Two areas are selected. Firstly, communication and teamwork, and secondly the difficult question of the appropriate use of drugs.

I have quoted from the work of several of my colleagues to whom I am grateful, in particular Dr Alistair Tulloch and Dr Julian Tudor Hart.

Though the problems are similar in all developed countries, the context of this presentation is the National Health Service in the United Kingdom.

DO GENERAL PRACTITIONERS FACE PROBLEMS IN CARING FOR THE ELDERLY?

Care of the elderly is a major and traditional concern of general practitioners. Many continue to care for them in traditional ways. But times are changing, and many GPs are finding their work-load increasing. Maybe the consultation and home-visit rates are steady or even falling, but the content of the consultation is often more intense, and the load of telephone calls, correspondence, and meetings is increasing.

This increased work-load is a reflection of a number of trends, which are listed below. Many of them are likely to increase in the next twenty years. They can be divided into factors within the practice – over which GPs may have some measure of control – and outside factors, both medical and social, to which general practice must adapt if it is to survive.

Factors for change within primary care

Increasing emphasis on caring for the elderly in the community.
The development of community hospitals.

Factors operating outside the practice

Medical

Fewer hospital beds (acute, geriatric, and psychiatric).
Shorter hospital inpatient stay.
Longer waiting lists for outpatients.
The 'silent epidemic' of dementia in the elderly (OHE 1979).

Social

An aging population.*
Fewer 'supporters' in a position to care for elderly relatives, because of smaller family size, social mobility, and more women at work.
Changes in expectations of care.
Decreased spending by local authorities on residential care of the elderly.

The factors listed all combine to put pressure on the primary care and community services, but the picture is not all black. There are several countervailing trends which are hopeful:

More health visitors attached to general practice.

Appointment of community psychiatric nurses, geriatric health visitors, 'catheter nurses', night nursing, etc.

Increased spending on equipment for disabled living at home.

Improved range of prescription items and nursing aids for the disabled (e.g. for incontinence).

Developing role of the practice nurse and practice manager.

Technological advance in managing disability (Wolff 1980) (see Chapter 9).

Hospital and local authority services are slow to react to changes in demand, so the load will inevitably fall on general practice and the community services. The time factor is against us, so we must move quickly to adapt, or face being overwhelmed by demand.

Each practice must approach this issue in the light of its own unique circumstances and make a ten- or twenty-year survival plan. How to make and implement plans is set out in more detail elsewhere (Pritchard 1981; Pritchard, Low, and Whalen 1982).

The first step is to accept that there is a problem and decide to do something

---

*In the past 20 years, the numbers over 65 have risen by one-third. They now constitute 15 per cent of the population and the numbers are still growing. The average age of the older generation is rising, so that by the end of the century the number aged 75 and over will have increased by about one-fifth, and the number aged 85 and over by one-half. Three-quarters of these will be women – many of whom will be on their own. (HMSO 1981 – Growing Older).

about it. The next, and much more difficult, steps are to make plans; motivate people to carry them out; implement the plans; then take a look to see what has been achieved and what to do next.

CAN PREVENTIVE MEASURES HELP?

Though prevention of diseases and disability related to aging must be considered one of the major challenges facing medicine today, it has not had the attention which, in my view, it deserves. The Royal College of General Practitioners has firmly espoused the cause of prevention, and set up four working parties (RCGP 1981a). One was concerned with the prevention of arterial disease, which has considerable implications for the elderly (RCGP 1981b). Apart from this the special problems of the people aged 75 and over were not stressed, though no doubt this omission will soon be remedied.

Many objectives for prevention could be considered,* and I have selected three to which general practitioners can make a major personal contribution:
Prevention of arterial disease.
Early diagnosis and treatment of disabling conditions.
Prevention of accidents.

Prevention of arterial disease

Myocardial infarcts, strokes, hypertension, and peripheral arterial disease carry a heavy mortality and morbidity. Much of the work-load falls on general practitioners.
Risk factors include:
Cigarette smoking.
High arterial blood pressure (over 90 diastolic 5th phase).
Diabetes.
Obesity and excess blood lipids.
Lack of exercise.
Excess salt in diet.
As well as causing over half the deaths over 65, arterial disease causes half the deaths under 65, and a considerable load of ill-health. The earlier we start preventive measures the more effective they will be, but better late than never.

General practitioners would find it difficult to influence all these risk factors, but a start can be made on cigarette smoking and hypertension.

Cigarette smoking

Health education programmes cannot easily compete with massive advertising of cigarettes, nor easily change long-established behaviour. This need not cause despair, as it is possible for general practitioners to have considerable influence

---

*See also Chapter 7.

on the smoking habits of their patients. For further ideas see Stott and Davis (1979), and Russell *et al.* (1979).

What practical steps can the general practitioner take?

1. Record smoking habits of all patients in the notes at their next attendance.
2. Draw the attention of patients with arterial disease to the risk of smoking. (Approximate doubling of mortality.)
3. Choose a suitable moment to recommend them strongly to give up smoking.
4. Reinforce the advice with booklets such as 'The Smokers Guide to Non Smoking'.*
5. Put patient in touch with self-help groups in neighbourhood.
6. Ask about smoking at follow-up visits, and encourage further effort.
7. Set an example in non-smoking!
8. Temper enthusiasm with sympathy.

Detection and treatment of hypertension

Much of the ethos of prevention has been concerned with keeping breadwinners alive and well. As a result the evidence about hypertension mostly relates to people up to the age of 65 (RCGP 1981*b*). However, Miall and Chinn (1973) showed clearly that arterial pressure reached its peak in 75. Julian Tudor Hart (1980) has an excellent chapter on arterial pressure in the elderly to which the reader is referred. Some of his conclusions (pp. 244–5) are paraphrased here:

There is good evidence that high arterial pressure causes strokes in those under 70.

There is little evidence that this applies in people over 70, or that treating hypertension in people over 70 is effective. †

The most effective way to treat hypertension in the elderly is to control it in middle age and maintain that control.

This suggests that screening for hypertension – already a desirable objective for general practice – should be rigorously pursued and, if resources allow, extended up to the age of 70, rather than stopping at 65.

How can this be done?

Hart (1980) has covered this topic very fully. I will describe only the essentials of a screening programme in general practice, based on his work.

Decisions will have to be taken which are listed:

Age range to be covered, e.g. 30–64 if resources are scanty, 20–64 (or 69) for full ascertainment.

---

*Obtainable free of charge from Health Education Council, 78 New Oxford Street, London, WC1A 1AH. (Or Local Health Education Unit.)
† This view may need to be modified in the light of recent trials.

Limits of blood pressure – 'three box system'

		Age 40–64*
A	For treatment	180+/105+
B	For observation after one year	155/90 to 179/104
C	For re-check after five years	<155/<90

or 'two box system in which B and C are combined in five-year check.

Method of screening – on attendance with notes flagged (see operational check-list, p. 204).

Or using age–sex register and postal reminders (much more costly, but better suited to computerization).

Will extra staff hours be needed for extra workload?† e.g. Clerk, Practice Nurse, Doctor.

Staff training and motivation needed.

Equipment needed – e.g. service existing sphygmomanometers, or buy new ones (mercury type preferred, at about £20 each). Will also need markers for notes:

Red – for all patients screened – say 1500
Green – for five years later – say 1500
Five other colours for each year (initially only
for 'observation' group) – say 100 of each.

How to obtain resources.

When to start.

When to assess results, and how.

A flow-chart to illustrate such a screening programme is shown in Fig. 11.1. A procedural check-list follows. These are only examples, and would need to be modified to suit local circumstances.

The decision whether to screen patients when they turn up, or undertake a much more elaborate method using the age–sex register to screen the whole practice is difficult. Cartwright and Anderson (1981) found that at all ages about one-fifth of patients did not consult their doctor in the previous year. For those aged 65–74 the proportion was about one-third. Thus a screening programme based on attending the surgery would cover two-thirds of the age

*For limits of blood pressure under the age of 40 see Hart (1980).

†Based on Hart's (1980) data, the numbers under treatment would be as follows:

Age 20–39 = 1.5 per cent. Age 40–64 = 7.5 per cent. Age over 64 = 4.5 per cent. The total number in a practice of 2500 would be about 70. The extra work-load can be set against Miall's (1973) estimate of 14 strokes prevented every ten years for every 10 000 patients screened. The possible reduction in mortality and morbidity from other forms of arterial disease, and link with antismoking education would be an additional bonus, but hard to quantify.

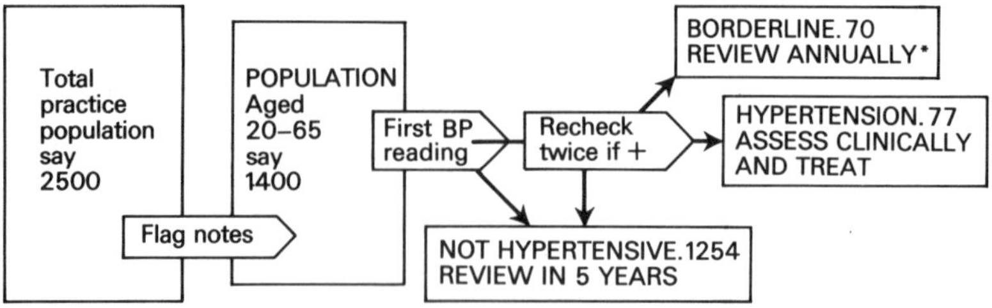

204 *Practical issues facing the general practitioner in caring for the elderly*

```
┌──────────┐  ┌──────────┐                        ┌─────────────────────┐
│ Total    │  │POPULATION│                        │BORDERLINE. 70       │
│ practice │  │Aged      │                        │REVIEW ANNUALLY*     │
│population│  │20–65     │ First BP    Recheck    ├─────────────────────┤
│ say      │  │say       │ reading     twice if + │HYPERTENSION. 77     │
│ 2500     │  │1400      │                        │ASSESS CLINICALLY    │
│          │  │          │                        │AND TREAT            │
└──────────┘  │          │                        └─────────────────────┘
      Flag notes          │
              │          │    ┌─────────────────────┐
              └──────────┘    │NOT HYPERTENSIVE.1254│
                              │REVIEW IN 5 YEARS    │
                              └─────────────────────┘
```

Fig. 11.1. Flow chart of hypertension screening plan. *If the 'three-box' system is not used, these patients would be regarded as 'not hypertensive' and reviewed after five years. (Based on Hart (1980) Appendix 1.)

groups at risk, and the proportion would increase with time. This would probably be the best option for those who do not have a computerized age–sex register.

Operational check-list for hypertension screening

Clerk

Go through all practice notes.

Put red 'flag' in all those aged 20–70 (or agreed age limits).

Receptionist

When patient attends, check if BP has been taken in past year.

If BP is less than 140/85 remove red flag and insert green flag colour coded to represent five years hence. (If in doubt refer to practice nurse.)

Remainder – ask practice nurse to see patient to check BP before seeing doctor, if time allows and patient agrees.

New patients – insert red flag and refer to nurse.

Practice nurse

Take blood pressure in accordance with procedure in Hart (1980), Appendix 4, pp. 249–30.

If 'normal', remove red flag and insert green flag (colour code = five years hence).

If 'borderline' remove red flag and replace with appropriate colour for next year.

If 'raised', repeat twice at about weekly intervals. If subsequent reading is normal, proceed as above.

If still 'raised':

    1. Check urine for protein, glucose, and blood and record in notes.

    2. Take blood for blood count, urea, creatinine, and electrolytes.

    3. Do ECG, or get one done.

    4. Enquire about smoking habits and record in notes. Counsel appropriately and give handouts.

    5. Check weight and record in notes.

6. Put blue sticker on outside of notes and remove red flag.
7. Refer patient and record to doctor.

Doctor
Take history, including family history.
Check smoking habits and counsel.
Examine weight, heart, lungs, ankles, peripheral pulses, carotids, fundi.
Check results of tests done by practice nurse and laboratory.
Negotiate treatment plan with patient, and start it.
Arrange follow-up (not exceeding three monthly).

Follow-up
Fail-safe recall system needed so that defaulting does not escape notice.
Receptionist
To send appointment to see:
Practice nurse who checks weight, BP, urine, and then see:
Doctor to re-check BP, adjust treatment, and make further follow-up appointment.

Review:
Clerk
At end of first calendar year, get out all notes which still have a red flag. Pass them to:
Practice nurse to check if normal BP has been recorded in past five years. If so, remove red flag and replace with appropriate colour for five years from date of reading.
If no record, or BP raised or borderline, refer notes to doctor to decide on postal request to attend, *or nurse* to visit, *or doctor* to visit or telephone.
Leave red flag in till patient attends.

Early diagnosis and treatment of disabling conditions

Ann Cartwright's figures just quoted indicate the reluctance, or inability of some older patients to visit their doctor, yet this is a group in which particular vigilance is needed to detect potentially disabling conditions which are treatable.

Geriatric screening

Some practices have tried to get round this difficulty by a 'geriatric screening' programme. In my own practice such a survey was done five years ago, and the general opinion of doctors, nursing staff, and patients was that it was worth doing. However, it was not properly evaluated.

Tulloch and Moore (1979) did a more detailed survey of a sample of patients aged 70 and over and this was evaluated and compared with a control group at the end of a two-year period. The survey revealed 144 previously undetected medical conditions in 145 patients. Sixty-seven per cent of the medical conditions were found to be manageable. Half were improved and half completely resolved. The surprising finding was that the case-control study over two years did not demonstrate any differences between the screened and unscreened patients in the prevalence of health problems. The screened group did, however, seem to have less pain, were less disabled and were independent for longer. There was some improvement in their morale and self-esteem.

Staff too can feel more confident that they have the measure of the level of disability among the elderly in their area.

Hannay (1979) in his monumental work on the 'symptom iceberg', showed that there was a substantial level of illness not brought to the notice of a doctor in people over 65, particularly in women.

Geriatric screening is one answer to the problem of unreported and untreated illness in the community, and a specimen proforma and procedures follow this section. Each practice must decide for itself whether to undertake this task, and make its own detailed objectives and plans. Much of the work is done by the health visitor and district nurse, so their enthusiasm is essential for success, as is the agreement of nursing management, and the laboratory service.

If a full sociomedical screening programme is not feasible, progress can be made on a narrower front by concentrating on certain major risk-factors. Hypertension screening has already been described. Musculoskeletal disorders are a major cause of loss of independence; and because of restricted mobility are more likely to go untreated. Other major risk-factors in the elderly are accidents; hypothermia and loss of vision and hearing. These could be included in a more restricted screening programme.

Involving the community

An alternative strategy is to raise the level of public awareness and involvement, so that the health care team has a larger and more responsive information base. Many voluntary organizations in the community such as the Red Cross, Women's Institutes, Townswomen's Guilds, Church organizations, and Women's Royal Voluntary Service already perform services for the elderly, and report any loss of independence or need for medical care – as indeed do postmen and milkmen. Age Concern has a co-ordinating role in voluntary services for the elderly. Self-help groups and older people's clubs, are all part of this very complex caring and alerting network.

Can the health team ensure that people working in the community are looking for key risk-factors as well as combating loneliness and isolation? Doctors and health visitors can talk and discuss these issues with clubs and local groups, and a slot for health problems of the elderly on local radio is particularly appropriate.

If the practice has a patient participation group or committee (RCGP 1981c) this can have a valuable function as a 'listening post' in the community, as well as actually providing services for the elderly such as surgery transport, prescription delivery, lunch clubs, etc.

Geriatric survey: procedures

Secretary

(a) Prepare list of all patients of each doctor over 70, or 75, from age/sex register or computer listing.

(b) Pass list to doctor who will delete any who are already under supervision, or known refusals.

(c) Fill in heading of proforma, attach to medical record, and pass to doctor at agreed rate (say four per week).

(d) Record entry to geriatric survey on list.

Doctor

(a) Complete section A with relevant medical diagnoses/problems.

(b) Pass to health visitor for action.

Health visitor

(a) Check medical record if necessary, e.g. hospital or social reports.

(b) Return record for filing.

(c) Complete social enquiry section B, from own records.

(d) If information missing, visit patient and complete section B.

(e) Pass proforma to district nurse for action.

District nurse

(a) Visit patient and explain purpose and nature of survey, request co-operation, and ensure that informed consent is given.

(b) Enquire about symptoms using the following repertoire:

Section C
1. Is your appetite normal?
2. Do you have indigestion or pain after meals?
   Do any foods upset your stomach?
3. Is your weight steady now, or have you lost any weight recently?
4. Do you have a cough? Do you cough up any sputum? Is it white, yellow, or bloodstained?
5. Do you have any chest pain? Where is it situated? Is it made worse by exertion, or cold weather?
6. Are you short of breath when you exert yourself? (e.g. hurrying, climbing stairs).
7. Are any of your joints painful?

8. Do you have to get up at night to pass water? Is it ever painful? Do you have any difficulty in holding your water? (e.g. when you cough or sneeze).
   Have you ever had blood in the water?
9. Do you go to the toilet to pass a motion every day? Are you constipated? Is passing a motion painful? Do you ever have diarrhoea? Have you noticed blood in your motions? Have you ever passed black motions like tar?
10. Have you had any bleeding from the back passage? (Females) Have you had discharge or bleeding from the front passage?
11. Have you any other symptoms or complaints? (Help patient to verbalize these).

Please comment if patient has difficulty understanding the questions, or does not give reliable answers, or is mentally confused.

Put X in column if any *positive* symptoms and specify details.

Section D: Physical checks*

1. Test vision with card at three metres, with glasses. Specify if one or both eyes faulty.
2. Check mouth and specify if dental caries, or inadequate dentures, from the point of view of function.
3. Check hearing by quiet speech with each ear covered in turn. Check for wax with auriscope.
4. Check neck veins for rise of jugular venous pressure above clavicle.
5. Check ankles for pitting oedema.
6. Check vibration sense in ankles; against tibial tuberosity and head of radius.
7. Examine feet for corns, callouses, and assess need for professional chiropody (instruct in home care of feet if relevant.)
8. Obtain urine specimen at time of interview and check by uristix and culture at laboratory.
   Arrange for later specimen to be collected using MSU technique (no Cetrimide).
9. Record blood pressure sitting. Take three readings and record.
10. Check weight on portable scales.
11. Take blood for:
    Haemoglobin
    ESR
    Urea and creatinine.

Record any other relevant observations.

*The district nurse will need the following equipment, and may need training in its use:
Vision testing card for use at three metres. Pen torch. Auriscope. Tuning fork. Blood pressure machine. Portable scales. Two bottles for urine sampling. Uristix or equivalent. 20 ml sterile syringe. Needle. EDTA and fluoride bottles.

Section E

Please list all tablets, capsules or medicine taken by patient, including self-medication. Complete column of number per day from patient's answer. When form complete, pass to secretary.

Secretary

Collect laboratory results and clip to proforma. Attach to medical record and pass to doctor for action. Arrange surgery appointment if mobile. Put on visiting list if not mobile.

Doctor
- (a) Check survey and laboratory results.
- (b) Visit patient
- (c) Examine heart, lungs, abdomen, and other systems if indicated.
- (d) Ask and record tobacco and alcohol intake.
- (e) Update problem list A.
- (f) Record action recommended and by whom.
- (g) Record review interval.
- (h) Discuss with health visitor or district nurse if needed.
- (i) Pass to secretary

Secretary
- (a) Pass messages about action.
- (b) Diary when action completed, or remind.
- (c) Diary review interval.
- (d) File proforma in medical record.

GERIATRIC SURVEY : PROFORMA

Name	Surname	Forenames	M.S.W.

Address: .... GP...............

.... HV...............

D of B....................

A. *Medical diagnoses/problems* (Dr to list)   *Date of diagnoses*
   1.
   2.
   3.
   4.
   5.
   6.

B. *1st Visit   Health visitor**   Date......................

   Accommodation: House/flat/bungalow/caravan/other
   Facilities:
   Social contacts/isolation:

Does impaired mental state affect independence?	YES/NO
Does poor motivation affect independence?	YES/NO
Does impairment of vision, speech or hearing affect independence	YES/NO

   Is patient INDEPENDENT for: Comments

Mobility indoors	YES/NO
Mobility outdoors	YES/NO
Dressing	YES/NO
Food	YES/NO
Toilet	YES/NO
Bathing	YES/NO
Household tasks	YES/NO
Finance	YES/NO

   Aids
   Treatments

---

*It is important that the health visitors' Social Enquiry form corresponds with the one she normally uses. These questions are taken from the form used by Oxfordshire Area Health Authority (Teaching).

C. **2nd Visit   District nurse**   Date......................
    Symptomatic enquiry   (Mark X if present)
    1. Poor appetite
    2. Indigestion
    3. Loss of weight
    4. Productive cough
    5. Substernal pain
    6. Short of breath
    7. Painful joints
    8. Abnormal micturition
    9. Difficulty with bowels or diarrhoea
    10. Rectal or vaginal bleeding
    11. Other symptoms – please list
       ....
       ....

D. *Physical checks*   (Mark X if present)
    1. Visual acuity (with glasses) (worse than 6/60)
                                    (worse than 6/18)
                                    6/18 or better)
    2. Dental problem
    3. Hearing loss (check with auriscope)
    4. Jugular venous pressure raised
    5. Oedema of ankles
    6. Vibration sense lost in feet
    7. Needs chiropody (examine feet)
    8. Urine (contains protein)
            (contains glucose)
            (MSU sent to lab.)
    9. Blood pressure (sitting)   (Systolic)
       Repeat if raised   (Diastolic (phase 5))
    10. Weight
    11. Blood taken for (FBC)
                       (ESR)
                       (Urea/creatinine)
    Other observations:
    ....
    ....

E. *List of current medication* (include self-medication)

Name of drug or medicine	Size or quantity	No. of times daily

F. *3rd Visit   Doctor*   Date......................
    Examine heart   normal/abnormal......................
    Examine lungs   normal/abnormal......................
    Examine abdomen   normal/abnormal......................
    Other systems indicated by questionnaire:
    ....
    ....
    Daily quantity smoked? ....
    Daily alcohol consumption? ....
    Doctor update problem list A.
    Action recommended: By whom?
    ....
    ....
    ....

    Review interval: .... months
                              .... years

Prevention of accidents

Accidents take a terrible toll in old age, particularly among women aged 75 and over.* We all know how often a fractured femur condemns a lively old lady to a life of pain and dependency – in spite of the undoubted advances in surgical care. Many of these accidents are preventable, so what can general practitioners do to prevent as many of them as possible? The responsibility falls squarely on the health visitor in her role as health educator, but all the team can join in and help. Joint discussions with the whole team can co-ordinate plans in which all can be involved.

Falls

The educative process can start when people retire. They can be encouraged to make their houses 'accident proof' by attention to carpets, stairs, lights, high cupboards, etc. A helpful booklet is published by the Royal Society for Prevention of Accidents entitled 'Safety in retirement' which contains a checklist of potential dangers in the home. (Making the home safe for grannies also helps to make it safe for young grandchildren who are known to be at greater risk when staying with grandparents.) The Health Education Council also has a good booklet on 'Safety in the home'.

If the general practitioner is alert to all the possible hazards in the home, he can use his persuasive powers to get something done. Preretirement education is another area in which general practitioners can use their knowledge and skills.

Many falls take place at night when the old person gets up to pass water. Postural hypotension may result in a syncopal attack and a fall. This is more likely if the patient is on sleeping tablets. Studies have shown that at least one fifth of women aged 75 and over are taking psychotrophic drugs. Often this habit started when they were bereaved, and it is open to question whether these drugs are helpful in the long term. Review of prescribing in the elderly will be discussed later. Other conditions causing elderly people to fall are discussed elsewhere.

Osteoporosis

The epidemiology of fractures in the elderly makes alarming reading. Aging normally produces a loss of skeletal tissue at a rate of 0.5 per cent per annum from the time of the menopause in women, and from the age of 60 in man. The results can be seen in Table 11.1.

Overall, at least 25 per cent of western women suffer at least one such fracture in their lives. Unfortunately, there is little agreement whether any attempt should be made to prevent this appalling level of suffering by drug

---

*Nearly three-quarters of 'all accidents other than motor vehicle accidents' at all ages, occur in females aged 75 and over, and for males the figure is a quarter. This represents over 4000 deaths per annum in England and Wales, and much disability (OPCS 1976).

Table 11.1. *Cumulative incidence of fractures with age* (from Nordin, C., 1978)

Fracture of	Incidence Women	Men
Lower forearm	15% by age 80	4% by age 80
Vertebrae	8% by age 80	4% by age 80
Femoral neck	10% by age 85	3% by age 85

therapy in later years. Possible treatment would include oral calcium and vitamin D; oral fluoride; cyclical oestrogen, or progestogen treatment in women; parenteral testosterone in men. The effectiveness of intervention would have to be established in large-scale trials before a programme on this scale could be undertaken. It would be costly, but the benefits could be very great.

Many doctors feel that their job is to treat the sick, and not to involve themselves in preventive programmes which cost money and time, and may divert them from their curative role. In this they have an ally in King Canute who did not act till it was too late. I would suggest that his modern counterpart could avoid trouble by looking up the tide tables!

Time and cost are valid objections. I hope that ways will be found to re-imburse doctors who undertake preventive work (Dr Hart suggests 100 per cent re-imbursement). The time burden will fall mostly on other staff, and will eventually relieve the load on the doctor.

WHAT ELSE CAN WE DO?

Developing team work and streamlining communications

I have argued earlier that general practitioners can expect a considerable increase in their work-load in the next ten or twenty years. A preventive approach will take time, and will not be enough to stem the tide of demand. Another option is to make the fullest use of other team members and to delegate. To do this requires an understanding of team work and a commitment to make a success of it. In addition, good communication procedures are needed, both within the practice and with outside agencies such as departments of geriatric medicine, social services, and voluntary bodies. Team work and communication are interdependent, so are considered together in this section.

Different teams for different tasks

A team is 'A group of people who have different contributions toward the achievement of a common goal'. Primary health care has a lot of different goals and performs a multiplicity of tasks. I have found it easier to consider the team at its simplest and most basic in order to understand its workings and make it successful.

An example may be helpful:

A woman patient aged 75 develops a stroke when living at home with her daughter. The doctor is called who diagnoses a Rt hemiplegia due to cerebral thrombosis. He asks the district nurse to visit to make a nursing assessment and give nursing care. She reports back to him what she has done and they discuss the treatment plan with the patient and her daughter. All agree that the patient should be nursed at home.

This is a team consisting of doctor, district nurse, patient, and supporter, which I have called the 'intrinsic' team (Pritchard 1981) as this is the basic unit of team care, involved in a task for an individual patient. As the task changes other members may join or leave, but the 'intrinsic' team continues to revolve aroung the patient as long as there is work to be done (see Fig. 11.2).

For the intrinsic team to function, each must know what the other is capable of – and not capable of. That is to say the roles and role-boundaries. These need not be rigid in a well-functioning team where there is flexibility in 'who does what'. Failure to define tasks and understand each other's job can lead to conflict, which is often put down to personality clashes when that is not the underlying cause.

TASK: Management of acute illness at home — The intrinsic team

SUPPORTER

PATIENT

GENERAL PRACTITIONER   COMMUNITY NURSE

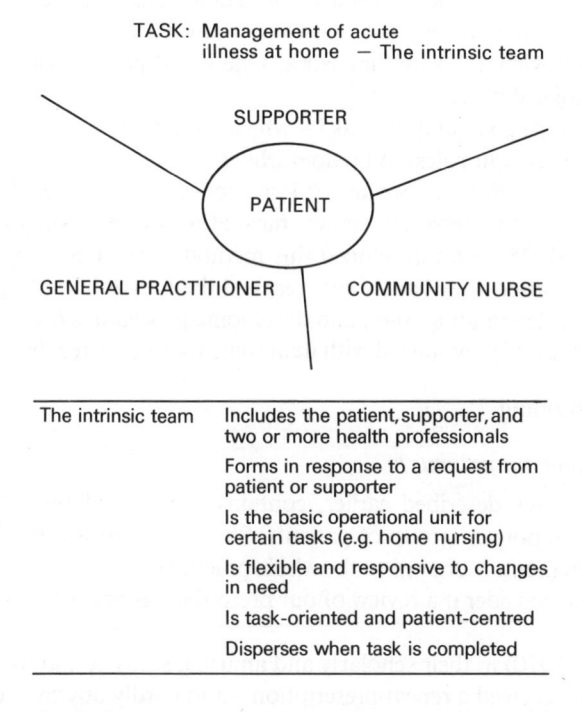

The intrinsic team	Includes the patient, supporter, and two or more health professionals
	Forms in response to a request from patient or supporter
	Is the basic operational unit for certain tasks (e.g. home nursing)
	Is flexible and responsive to changes in need
	Is task-oriented and patient-centred
	Disperses when task is completed

Fig. 11.2. The home nursing team. An example of the 'intrinsic' team.

The other prerequisite for successful team working is to have good working procedures agreed by all. Meeting daily over coffee is a good start. There must be clear message-passing methods such as a day book in which all messages are written down, and which the secretary checks daily to ensure all messages have been picked up.

Each general practitioner and attached district nurse would probably share about ten active cases. It is helpful for them to have regular meetings (say every six weeks) in which these cases are reviewed. This is a different sort of team, without patients or supporters, consisting of two (or more) professionals, taking a regular look at their mutual case load, and at their working procedures. In my experience these meetings are brief, brisk, and popular. Similar meetings can be undertaken with health visistors, practice nurses or receptionists. In each case a different *function* of primary care is discussed, e.g. home nursing, prevention, administration, etc. I have therefore called them 'functional' teams. For further details of their working see Pritchard (1981), which also has some ideas for team-building.

Developing team working

Attaching nursing staff to general practice is crucial to team working, as is frequent contact, and – if possible – shared premises. But throwing them together does not make them into a team. They have to build this up by a deliberate educational process. The most important part of it is to be prepared to take time to review the way they work. One bit of good advice is to tackle problems in a logical order.

First: What is the goal, and the task? – why are we here?
Second: What are our roles? Who does what?
Third: What procedures do we agree? How do we do things here?
Fourth and last: Interpersonal relationships. How do we get on together?

Rubin *et al.* (1975), who developed this method in the USA found that by working in that order, they hardly ever reached the fourth item. Experience of sharing tasks, understanding roles, and developing procedures together ensured good relationships; if they started with item four, they never reached the task!

Review of prescribing

Are we poisoning our patients?

The geriatric survey described earlier, contains a review of prescribing for a small but very important group of patients. Should this review be extended to all our elderly patients – or even to the whole practice?

First we must consider if a review of our prescribing is needed, or is it beyond reproach?

Balint *et al.* (1970) in their scholarly and amusing study found that a quarter of their sample received a repeat prescription – and hardly anything else – from their doctors. But then it would seem that they had no recognizable illness!

'detailed clinical studies revealed that the so-called successful or "peaceful" repeat prescriptions had hardly anything to do with rational therapy based on a sensible diagnosis'. Doctors were colluding to keep the peace. It was difficult to get out of this trap.

There have been a number of epidemiological studies of prescribing with roughly comparable findings, but I will in particular quote Murdoch (1980). He found that the bulk of total prescribing was for the elderly, and this was mostly for continued items. Females received more prescriptions than males. There was a steep rise after 75 in prescribing of diuretics, and in males, hypnotics and tranquillizers. In females the rise for the last two started at 65. In patients 65 years and over, 59 per cent of prescriptions were for long-term repeats. If we are to review prescribing over 65, the greatest impact could be made by first studying the largest groups, i.e. long-term repeat prescriptions, and concentrating on those drugs which we think may be prescribed unnecessarily.

Tulloch (1981) listed the following for special review:
tranquillizers
hypnotics
antidepressants
diuretics
digoxin
antacids
hypotensive drugs.

He found that 10 per cent of prescriptions for patients aged 65 and over were thought to be unnecessary, and 28 per cent equivocal. These accounted for 29 per cent of prescribing costs. These figures can be regarded as an underestimate, because he had about half the average number of patients aged 65 and over in his practice, and his prescribing costs were 36 per cent below the national average before the review.

Repeat prescription cards

Many authors in this field have stressed the importance of the repeat prescription card held by the patient. If the format could be agreed with the local geriatricians, it could become a co-operation card to bridge the chasm between geriatricians' beliefs about what the patient is (or should be) taking, and reality. Baxendale *et al.* (1978) have pioneered this approach.

GPs do not need to seek out their patients in this kind of review. The prescriptions are regularly presented to them for signing. They need to approach each one critically. It is a help to have a polite letter duplicated to ask patients to attend for review, rather than go on with repeat prescriptions indefinitely. Those wishing to set up a repeat prescription system would do well to consult Drury (1981) for details.

For an excellent review of prescribing for the elderly in general practice see Knox (1980), in which appears the quotation: 'How is one to teach (and learn) the art of *non-prescribing*?'.

In conclusion

In this brief chapter I have only been able to select a few areas for attention. There are many others which may seem as pressing – and indeed may be more so – for every practice is different. However, we cannot do everything at once, and an essential lesson in managing general practice is to select objectives of high priority *which are achievable* and get started straight away.

I hope that the objectives which I have touched upon – hypertension screening – geriatric survey – prevention of accidents – team development – improved communications – improved prescribing are achievable and worthwhile. They all depend upon efficient management and teamwork within the practice, as well as good relationships with geriatric services and community physicians which is the theme of this book.

12 Terminal care in the home
Roy Spilling

INTRODUCTION

One's own home can be the best but also the worst place to die. Many factors influence the outcome, but the key role in determining the adequacy of care is given to the general practitioner, who provides all the medical care in the last year of life to three-tenths of the population, and looks after the medical needs of most of the other seven-tenths prior to hospital admission. Generally, he is in the best position to co-ordinate the care of the hospital, district nursing and social services, and to communicate the requirements of the patient to the family and those most able to help.

WHO DIES AT HOME?

Diagnostic groups

The common causes of death are shown in Table 12.1. It is of interest to note that in malignant disease, when death tends to be expected, two-thirds die in hospital; whereas in circulatory disease, when death is often relatively sudden, a half die at home. Those suffering from unusual (? interesting) diseases are most likely to die in hospital.

Table 12.1. *Place and cause of death in England and Wales* 1969

Diagnostic groups	Percentage of total deaths (579,378)	Percentage in each group dying in Hospital	Home
Circulatory	52	52	48
Neoplastic	20	63	37
Respiratory	15	65	35
Accidents	4	53	47
Other	9	80	20

After Cartwright *et al.* (1973).

The trend since 1969 has been for a reduction in the number of deaths at home, a trend in which deaths from cancer mirror the other causes of death (Table 12.2).

Many reasons for this trend may be cited:
1. The increasing proportion of our population over 65 years of age (Table 12.3) results in:

Table 12.2. *Deaths at home as a percentage of ages of all, and of cancer deaths*

	All deaths	At home (%)	Cancer deaths	At home (%)
1965	549 000	38	107 000	37
1974	585 000	31	123 000	31

From Registrar General's Statistical Review of England and Wales 1976.

Table 12.3. *The elderly population of the UK (thousands)*

	1951	1971	1975
Men			
65–74	1600	2000	2161
75+	700	800	871
Total	2300	2800	3032
Women			
60–74	3500	4500	4592
75+	1100	1800	1911
Total	4600	6300	6483
All over retirement age as percentage of total population	13.6	16.3	17.0

From Central Statistical Office 1976 Social Trends No. 7. HMSO, London.

2. An increasing percentage living alone (Table 12.4), and therefore unable to care for themselves.

3. The increased mobility of the population has reduced the likelihood of children living nearby. The Age Concern survey (1974) showed that 40 per cent of the elderly did not have children living within one hour's distance. Even those who had children nearby seemed worried about imposing on them.

Table 12.4. *The elderly population living alone in private households in the UK (percentages)*

	1951	1971
Men		
65–74	6.5	10.9
75+	10.5	17.7
All elderly men (percentage)	7.7	13.0
Women		
60–74	15.6	27.0
75+	23.1	37.5
All elderly women (percentage)	16.8	30.0

From Central Statistical Office 1973 Social Trends No. 4. HMSO, London.

Who dies at home? 221

Talbe 12.5. *Who do the elderly live with? UK 1973–4 (percentages)*

Spouse	41
Married children	7
Unmarried daughter	5
Unmarried son	7
Grandchildren	4
Other relatives (65 or over)	4
Other relatives (65 or under)	3
Non-relatives	3
Alone	26

From Age Concern (1974). *The attitudes of the retired and elderly.* London.

4. More of the wives of married children had full or part-time employment which made the undertaking of nursing duties a difficult task.

5. Attitudes, too, within a family make it more difficult for an elderly dying person to find acceptance. Contemporary teenagers challenge the traditional authority of the elders.

6. Public expectation that hospital is the appropriate place to die has increased over the years, possibly because a reduction of infant mortality rates has made death itself a rarer experience in our western society.

Degree of warning

One death in ten is sudden and unexpected. That statistic, however, implies that in nine out of ten of our patients some degree of preparation for death is possible. A terminal illness is not always easy to define, but it can best be described as the illness in which the doctor becomes aware that death is inevitable, and turns his attention from cure to palliation. The aim of treatment then becomes the relief of symptoms rather than the removal of the cause. The duration of such terminal illness, in most instances, lasts from a few days to several months. This time presents the GP with one of his most demanding challenges – the opportunity to 'treat' death.

Restrictions in the last year of life

Mobility is affected to different extents and for different durations. Two-thirds of our patients will be restricted inside or outside the house for more than three months, and one-fifth of these will be bedridden or mainly confined to bed. This restriction of mobility is much more likely to be found in the elderly

Symptom control

Principles

Assessment It is important to (i) *Listen,* firstly, to the patient to find out which symptoms are predominant in his mind. What may seem to be trivial may have exaggerated importance to a dying patient. Secondly, to the relatives. The patient may put up a good face for his few minutes with the doctor. (ii) *Question,* specifically about pain. It is the commonest symptom of patients dying of cancer, and would appear to be unrelieved in nearly 50 per cent of those dying at home and 20 per cent of those dying in hospital (Parkes 1978). GPs are not unskilled in treating pain, but their patients appear to be particularly adept at concealing their sufferings from them. It is important, therefore, to ask supplementary questions, e.g. whether activity is limited, or sleep disturbed by, pain.

Diagnosis A particular symptom may have many different causes, and it is important to establish the most likely cause before commencing treatment.

Treatment

Explanation Fear accelerates symptoms, and treatment should begin with a simple explanation of cause and expectation of treatment to both patient and his relatives. Opportunity should be given for questions to be asked.

Simple remedies Local treatment of the pain from pressure areas, or the pruritus associated with jaundice is to be preferred to systemic therapy.

Drugs If drugs are used, then careful advice may ensure the addition of beneficial side-effects, e.g. the suppression of the respiratory centre by morphine in terminal dyspnoea. Note should be taken of the likely duration of action to determine frequency of dosage. Monitoring is important to ensure efficiency and also to assess the side-effects of treatment.

The doctor himself As it becomes obvious to the patient and his relatives that death is near, visits from the doctor become more important. Although he may himself feel powerless, his visible support helps all those concerned. The importance of touch also should not be underestimated. A quiet vigil holding the patient's hand conveys understanding and a willingness to share something of the suffering of the family.

Specific symptoms

Pain

The sensation of pain may be modified in the following ways:

Modification of the pathological process Deep irradiation, chemotherapy, or hormone treatment may be used by specialist colleagues. Recent evidence has implicated prostaglandin PGE_2 in producing the pain of osseous metastases. Aspirin and other non-steroidal anti-inflammatory preparations inhibit prostaglandin synthetase and therefore relieve pain through this mechanism as well as by increasing pain threshold.

Elevation of pain threshold Table 12.6 lists factors which alter the threshold above which pain is felt. Analgesic medication is one of the most effective methods of raising pain threshold. It is important to prevent pain by regular adequate dosage of the appropriate drug in the most convenient form. This will

Table 12.6. *Factors affecting pain threshold*

Threshold lowered	Threshold raised
Discomfort	Relief of symptoms
Insomnia	Sleep
Fatigue	Rest
Anxiety	Sympathy
Fear	Understanding
Anger	Diversion
Sadness	Elevation of mood
Depression	
Mental isolation	Analgesics
Introversion	Anxiolytics
Past experience	Antidepressants

After Twycross. from Saunders (1978).

usually mean four-hourly doses. Oral preparations are preferred wherever possible, and liquids are easier to manage than tablets. The choice of drug will be determined by the intensity of pain (Table 12.7). Oral morphine is as effective as oral diamorphine, and can be dispensed on its own in chloroform water, allowing individual requirements to dictate the dose in each 5 ml solution. If oral medication is not possible, morphine suppositories may be used which are equipotent with the oral form. However, if opiates have to be given by injection, the greater solubility of diamorphine makes it preferable to morphine, and the oral doses of both drugs should be halved for similar pain relief.

Interruption of pain pathways Specialized pain clinics may offer chemical or surgical nerve blocks for those whose pain is unrelieved by drugs.

Table 12.7. *Choice of analgesic preparation*

Type of pain	Drug	
Mild	Non-narcotic	Aspirin
		Paracetamol
Moderate	Weak narcotic	Codeine
		Di-hydro codeine
		Dextropropoxyphene
		Pentazocine
		Pethidine
Severe	Intermediate narcotic	Dipipanone
		Papaveratum
Very severe	Potent narcotics	Morphine
		Diamorphine
		Levallorphan
		Phenazocine
Overwhelming	Potent narcotics *and* anxiolytics, e.g.	Diazepam
		Chlorpromazine

From Twycross and Ventafridda (1980).

Immobilization Referral to orthopaedic surgeons should be considered for pathological fractures, as internal fixation should reduce the need for prolonged bed rest.

Adjuvant therapy Potent analgesics invariably have side-effects which may need an additional drug to counteract. *Laxatives* will usually be required with opiates, as will *anti-emetics,* such as chlopromazine (slightly sedative) or prochlorperazine (less sedative). The traditional use of cocaine to counteract the sedation of opiates has been largely dropped as tolerance appears to develop in a few days. *Corticosteroids* are often used where a large tumour mass causes pressure symptoms. A *diuretic* will also help in this situation. Steroids will also usually help the lethargy and depression of hypercalcaemia, e.g. Prednisone 10 mg t.d.s. Other non-specific uses of steroids are to improve appetite, to reduce fever, to enhance well-being, and to increase strength.

Sleeplessness

The benzodiazepines, e.g. Nitrazepam 5 mg are most commonly prescribed and have a useful anxiolytic action. Shorter-acting Temazepam or even shorter Triazolam are less likely to produce hang-over sedation.

Breathlessness

This is a difficult problem to treat and has many causes. Diuretics will improve the dyspnoea of heart failure, and bronchodilators may help if there is reversible airways obstruction. Steroids should be tried if there is neoplastic pressure on a bronchus. Heroin will reduce the intense discomfort when there is marked tachypnoea in the terminal patient.

Cough

Steam may be all that is needed to treat a spasmodic cough. Cough can be usefully controlled with 10 ml of Codeine linctus BPC or Methadone linctus (2 mg per 5 ml) 10 ml. This, of course, will be unnecessary if heroin is being prescribed for pain relief, which is in itself an effective cough suppressant.

Nausea and vomiting

If the cause is intracranial, Cyclizine (50–100 mg four hourly) will depress the emetic centre. If the patient is also anxious, it is best controlled by Prochlorperazine 5 mg, or Chlorpromazine 25 mg, which as mentioned before can be combined with an opiate mixture. Metoclopramide (10 mg) may be given two or three times daily, before food, if the cause is due to overstimulation of the bowel. This will also help nausea and vomiting of chemical origin. An additional cause of nausea and vomiting in terminal malignancy is hypercalcaemia which occurs in over 10 per cent of cases. A high fluid intake, steroids, and daily divided doses of effervescent phosphate tablets (1–3 g per day) i.e. 2–6 tablets of Phosphate-Sandoz per day will improve the situation in the majority of patients.

Constipation

Constipation is an extremely common problem in the terminally ill, and is often aggravated by the medication being taken for pain relief. Adequate fluids and stool softeners such as Dioctyl sulphosuccinate (Dioctyl-Medo) can be prescribed in syrup form. Bulk laxatives such as Celevac, Isogel, or Normacol will also help. Colonic stimulants such as bisacodyl (Dulcolax) may be used. Glycerine suppositories may be required and, of course, an occasional or even regular phosphate enema may be necessary.

Urinary incontinence

This, once infection has been excluded, might be helped by the use of Emepronium Bromide (Cetiprin) 200 mg. t.d.s., with 400 mg at night. It may, however, be necessary to resort to incontinence appliances or pads.

Confusion

Confusion at night may respond to Chloral as a hypnotic, or Chlormethiazole (Heminevrin) in a dose of 1 g. Daytime restlessness and confusion can be treated by Haloperidol to 15 mg t.d.s. or Thioridazine (Melleril) up to 50 mg t.d.s.; but watch must be made for parkinsonian side-effects. Chlormethiazole syrup, up to 10 ml t.d.s. (250 mg per 5 ml) may be used as an alternative if these occur, but will be more sedative.

Anxiety/depression

Alongside these physical and mental symptoms, the patient suffers the emotional symptoms of adjusting to the realization of dying. Hinton has shown that two-thirds of dying patients know they are dying, and are, in their own way, coming to terms with the loss of everything that is familiar. Dr Elizabeth Kubler-Ross in her book entitled *On death and dying* has shown the various phases through which dying patients pass. Denial, anger, bargaining, depression, and acceptance are not necessarily followed through sequentially, and many patients will move from one to another at different phases in their terminal illness. Depression as a symptom may initially best be treated by an open-ended discussion rather than by drugs. However, thare are a few patients who will benefit from tricyclic antidepressant therapy in their terminal illness. Others will be helped by the benzodiazepines (e.g. Diazepam 5 mg t.d.s.). Most of these symptoms, physical, mental and emotional are more severe in younger people than in the elderly.

A special mention ought to be made of the problem of children dying at home. Drs Chapman and Goodall have written helpfully of symptom control in this age group. A child's insight is often greater than an adult's but is expressed differently. Dr Bluebond-Langer's excellent study confirms the ability of children to behave in ways expected of them by the adult world, at the same time as persuing frank discussions with their peers. If talking about death makes their parents cry, they avoid it; for they are more concerned to have their mother and father with them than to have an accurate prognosis. Dying at home allows the maximum of familiar security for the child, and provides for the parents the optimum opportunity to express their care in nursing. Yet few children with gloomy prognoses are discharged from hospital to die at home. Recent interest in hospice support care for families with dying children is an encouraging sign.

WHO CARES?

Ninety per cent of patients dying in their homes are cared for by relatives, and 10 per cent by friends and neighbours. Most men dying are cared for by their wives, and most women dying are cared for by their daughters. The district nurse will be involved in the home care of the majority, but there are other sources of care which are listed in the next section. Nearly all patients dying either at home or in hospital are visited in their last year of life by the general practitioner, and he is therefore in a favoured position to assess the type of medical help needed by each particular patient and to enlist the help of the district nurse to make an assessment of nursing needs.

The bulk of home nursing falls on the relatives (Table 12.5) who themselves may not be well. Fourteen per cent of those dying at home with cancer, for example, are entirely looked after by relatives over the age of 70. The patient's symptoms which most trouble the relatives are in order of frequency: disturbance of sleep, incontinence of urine, restriction of social life, immobility, and faecal incontinence. The relatives' needs can best be summed up in one word – help! It is the GP's task to co-ordinate the various helps available.

THE GP AS CO-ORDINATOR

Aids

The relatives supplying the majority of nursing care will need to know where various aids can be obtained: walking sticks, Zimmer frames, urinals, bed pans, commodes, incontinence pads (or incontinence laundry, if available), sheepskin rugs and bootees, ripple mattresses. Most of these can be borrowed from the Red Cross or are available from the District Nursing Services.

Community Health Services

The district nurse

The district nurse should be involved in the care of the patient and the relatives. Traditionally her particular skills are in making the patient comfortable and clean, and tending to pressure sores, as well as supplying any form of medical treatment required. She can also involve the help of the bathing aids, but her expertise is in assessing nursing needs. Opportunities, however, at the bedside for listening have provided her with a counselling role which many patients use in preference to talking to a doctor.

The health visitor

The health visitor can advise the relatives of the services available, and is particularly skilled in the needs of the elderly and the care of dependent children. She can be invaluable in sharing the care of bereaved families with the GP.

The domiciliary occupational therapist

The domiciliary occupational therapist can provide help with modifications to the home, or provision of gadgets to make daily living (while dying) easier.

Voluntary support

Meals-on-wheels

Meals-on-wheels can provide a daily weekday hot meal, which may not be appreciated by the terminally ill, but will be by their elderly caring relatives.

Community care assistants

Community care assistants can make the life of the caring relative easier by helping in many different practical ways, e.g. shopping, or collecting prescribed items from the chemist.

Organizations

Organizations run under the auspices of the Church, Fish Neighbourhood scheme, or other body can also provide practical help. Such a scheme might provide 'night sitters' for dying patients.

The local clergy

The local clergy ought to be involved in providing comfort to both the patient and their relatives; families in such a situation are often slow to call in a priest, feeling that to do so is an admission that death is near. The family doctor should make a point of asking if such spiritual help would be welcomed.

Voluntary agencies for bereavement counselling

CRUSE the organization for widows and their children 260 Sheen Rd, Richmond, Surrey, tel. 01-940-4818. This organization uses 'professional' volunteers, e.g. social workers and clergy, and small self-help groups of 6–12 widows who meet regularly for support.

The Compassionate Friends, c/o Mrs Joan Wills, 50 Woodways, Watford, Herts., tel. Watford 24279. This self-help group is for parents who have lost a child.

The Samaritans, Church of St. Stephens, Walbrook, London EC4. This national organization through its telephone service offers immediate help at all times for people in trouble. Although used only by a small number of bereaved people, it offers a 'befriending service' for those tempted to suicide or despair.

Interval admissions

Local hospital services

Local hospital services can provide both day and holiday care in geriatric or continuing care units, arranged through the GP. The Hospice movement has contributed greatly to the welfare of the terminally ill. Hospices, traditionally charitable foundations often under the auspices of a religious order, together with the Marie Curie Memorial Foundation Homes, have provided a model which the NHS has followed. There are now 30–40 operating units in the UK run by the NHS. The building of many of them has been funded by the National Society for Cancer Relief and local charities. Several operate a day-care service for the terminally ill, and some are experimenting with a home-care service usually based on a continuing care unit.

The social services

The social services through their social workers have the skills to help people come to terms with their situation; and where possible, to alter their environment so as to improve the quality of life to the very end. For a variety of reasons, social worker involvement is frequently seen as crisis intervention and often comes too ineffectively too late. In the early stage of a terminal illness, a short term admission or day care at a Part III local authority home may be arranged to give the relatives a rest. Social workers do have much to offer the bereaved with their family casework training.

Extra nursing

Despite all the available help, home care may break down because of repeated disturbed nights, and the physical demands of a heavy bedfast patient. Caring for a terminally ill patient is a twenty-four-hour, seven-day-a-week, task for the family, yet most of the available services close down at night (or at weekends or bank holidays). The family doctor, acting on his own or with colleagues in a group practice, provides a service which does not close down, and a telephone call to a familiar person can be immensely reassuring to the family in the hours of darkness. This is of course assuming that he is already visiting the family regularly, rather than only when asked to do so.

'Twilight' (7–10 p.m.) nursing calls can be arranged through the district nursing service.

Nursing agencies, e.g. BUPA provide a private nurse 'bank' which provides 24-hour nursing cover and which operates a 10 p.m. to 8 a.m. night shift. Other agencies can provide SRN SEN psychiatric or auxiliary nurses at different rates of pay.

Charities such as the Marie Curie Foundation (124 Sloane Street, London SW1X 9 RF, tel. 01 730 9157) can provide extra nursing services for cancer patients in twelve-hour shifts from 8 p.m. Four kinds of nurse/attendant are recruited by the Foundation (i) SRN, (ii) SEN, (iii) auxiliary, and (iv) aide or sitter. It should be possible to arrange through the nursing officer for the Health Authority, the particular type of help required.

THE GP AS A COMMUNICATOR

The emotional symptoms experienced by the terminally ill are shared by their relatives. They, too, will show denial, anger, bargaining, depression and acceptance. The task of seeing through the denial of both relative and patient to make an accurate assessment of symptoms is not easy, as witnessed by the apparent poor pain control in terminal care at home. The patient's relatives' expectations of what must be suffered as death approaches are more influenced by their own childhood recollections of grandparents' deaths than by any knowledge of current therapeutics. Anxiety heightens awareness of pain: fear grows on uncertainties. This fear experienced by the dying has been analysed by Kastenbaum and Aisenberg. There are at least, three areas of concern:

Symptoms, particularly pain, may be uppermost in the mind. It is important to spend time in finding out the main worry and to explain an appropriate planned treatment programme.

Spiritual issues, such as fear of judgement, are often present even in patients who adopt a non-religious stance. The help of the clergy is invaluable.

Abandonment and loss. This can lie behind an unwillingness in the elderly to consider hospital admission. For them, too, the geriatric unit may have the image of the 'workhouse'. But death does sever human relationships, and time spent with the patient and his relatives allowing them to express their feelings often to each other through the listener can be profoundly comforting both to the dying and living. This demands of the doctor and the caring team a willingness to be open about the diagnosis and prognosis to the patient: an exacting task for which doctors, health visitors, and nurses will need their own support systems: e.g. regular meetings when death and bereavement can be discussed.

REASONS FOR HOSPITAL ADMISSION

A hospital admittance in terminal illness may be the deliberate choice of the patient, his family, or the medical team supervising the final weeks of life. This may be to a general hospital, continuing care unit, or to a community hospital where the GP can continue to care for both patient and family.

There are many reasons for hospital admission:

Nerve block treatment may require admission but specialist pain-relief centres are skilled in outpatient techniques.

Local or regional radio- or chemotherapy are only available in hospitals, but admission may not be necessary.

Items of equipment such as water-beds, hoists, etc. may not be readily available for home nursing.

Four-hourly injections may be difficult to administer in a patient's home, although well-motivated relatives can often be taught to give intramuscular drugs. Only a very small number of patients, however, cannot be managed with oral medication until the last few hours.

The majority of admissions in terminal illness, however, are required to give respite to an exhausted or frightened family, or where the community support has, for one reason or another, broken down. In these circumstances patients often spend a comparatively short time in hospital; a quarter of the admissions to St. Luke's Sheffield, die within three days. These may best be considered as failure of home care.

Only a third of admissions are for symptomatic relief, and severe pain is the commonest problem referred to hospital, but intractable vomiting or bleeding nearly always necessitates hospital care.

Other reasons for failure of home care include the need for nursing procedures such as injections, attention to pressure sores and mouth care, which if demanded by all the terminally ill patients at home, might increase the district-nursing load beyond the ability of the limited present level of staffing to cope.

This need for hospital referral of a terminally ill patient indicates another duty of the general practitioner, who aims to give the dying at home that which they and their relatives wish. As well as co-ordinating existing services, he must seek to create new ones for his own practice area, which might avoid admission to hospital for some patients. A rota of nurses for night injections, or of volunteers as night sitters would be two examples. He must also be prepared to step outside of his usual clinical role to attempt what few of us have the courage to do: to campaign vigorously for improved services. More district nurses would reduce the demand on expensive hospital beds at a time of economic hardship in the National Health Service. Yet the last ten years has shown expensive capital commitment to Terminal Care Units with little increase in the number of district nurses. The continuing care unit bed should not be seen as the norm for dying patients, but rather as an intensive therapy bed, for the staff:patient ratio can be 1:1. Such facilities should make them centres of excellence where research and teaching can inform the generalists in hospital and district services of the best methods of managing the dying patient and his family.

THE GP AS CERTIFIER

A family doctor is used to issuing certificates – of fitness to drive, attend college, take part in certain sports, of unfitness to work, of eligibility for all kinds of benefit, etc. One of the most important he issues is the death certificate to the grieving relative – the 'proof' for them that death can no longer be denied.

The final vigil at the bedside may be as important for a family doctor to share as attendance at the birth of a new member. It is certainly kindness to leave one's home phone number with the family and to be willing to attend at any hour to certify death. Despite the recent debate as to the criteria for the diagnosis of death, the GP supervising the terminal illness of one of his patients will not find it difficult to state that death has occurred. He should, however, not accept absence of respiration alone as confirming death, but should examine the fundi for 'trucking' of the vessels indicating stasis of the circulation. Rather than asking the relatives to call at the surgery for the death certificate, it is easy to carry a blank in one's bag, which can be signed and given to the family when certifying death. The stub in the certificate book can then be filled in later. Part I of a blank cremation form can be completed if requested, and left with the family at the same time for the second doctor to visit and complete Part II.

THE GP AS A COUNSELLOR

Although coming last in this chapter, the work of grieving begins for the surviving family with the news that death is inevitable. The emotional reactions of denial, anger, depression, and acceptance will be experienced not necessarily sequentially before the moment of death. A long stressful terminal illness may allow most of the grief work to be done by the survivors before death, so that the passing itself can really be a 'happy release'.

For the majority, however, the fact of death will dawn slowly. A few days of numbness, often terminated by the funeral, will lead to the characteristic phase of pining, in which pangs of severe anxiety are experienced. These are most frequent and severe usually within 5–14 days of bereavement, but tail-off later. They can, however, be revived when the memory is jogged and the lost person brought into mind. During this time, much of the activity of the bereaved can be understood as a searching process. The dead relative may be 'seen' or 'heard' or 'felt' and even talked to, and these experiences are usually comforting. It is important to reassure the grieving that they are not becoming insane when having these hallucinations, and that they should expect them to diminish with time. The anger of grief is often felt against the medical profession, but an understanding listening GP can help that particular breach to heal.

Bereavement visiting is best timed after the funeral when family and social supports tend to disappear. Another important occasion is the anniversary of the death.

The dividing line between normal and pathological grief is not clear, but extreme expressions of guilt or the delay of onset of pining beyond two weeks would favour medical intervention. The development of symptoms in the bereaved identical to those experienced by the dying relative indicates abnormal grieving.

For normal grief, drugs should not be prescribed, as a pattern of 'pill-taking' may be initiated, and the grief reaction may be prolonged. Relatives should be allowed to talk through the terminal illness and express their feelings in an atmosphere of understanding and support. Visits from the GP, health-visitors, nurses, and social workers encourage the bereaved to accept that mourning is a normal process, and an integral part of living.

Involvement of the voluntary agencies for bereavement counselling may be extremely supportive. The GP who knows his patients well, may be able to link up people who have been through similar expreriences and so create therapeutic groups.

The care of the dying at home is a very demanding but also rewarding part of the family doctor's task. The thirteenth century prayer of St. Francis illustrates an attitude which those involved in terminal care would do well to follow . . .

> Lord, make me an instrument of your health;
> Where there is sickness, let me bring cure;
> Where there is injury . . . aid;
> Where there is suffering . . . ease:
> Where there is sadness . . . comfort;
> Where there is despair . . . hope;
> Where there is death . . . acceptance and peace;
> Grant that I may not so much seek
> > to be justified, as to console;
> > to be obeyed, as to understand;
> > to be honoured, as to love;
> For it is in giving ourselves, that we heal;
> It is in listening that we comfort;
> And in dying, that we are born to eternal life.

Appendix 1. Useful addresses

Abbeyfield Society: 35a High Street, Potters Bar, Hertfordshire EN6 5DL.
Tel. Potters Bar (77) 43371

Abbeyfield Society: Northern Ireland Regional Council: Bryson House,
28 Bedford Street, Belfast B12 7BG.
Tel. Belfast (0232) 44660

Age Concern (England): Bernard Sunley House, 60 Pitcairn Road, Mitcham,
Surrey CR4 3LL.
Tel. 01 640 5431

Age Concern (Scotland): 33 Castle Street, Edinburgh EH2 3DN.
Tel. Edinburgh (031) 556 5000

Age Concern (Wales): 1 Park Grove, Cardiff CF1 3BJ.
Tel. Cardiff (0222) 371821

Age Concern (Northern Ireland): 128 Great Victoria Street, Belfast 2.
Tel. Belfast (0232) 45729

Alzheimer's Disease Society: c/o Neuropathology Department,
Radcliffe Infirmary, Oxford OX2 6HE.
Tel. Oxford (0865) 49891 ext. 815

Anchor Housing Association: Oxenford House, 13/15 Magdalen Street,
Oxford OX1 3BP.
Tel. Oxford (0865) 722261

British Red Cross Society: 9 Grosvenor Crescent, London SW1X 7EJ.
Tel. 01 235 5454

Counsel and Care for the Elderly: 131 Middlesex Street, London E1 7JF.
Tel. 01 621 1624

Crossroads Care Attendant Scheme Trust: 11 Whitehall Road, Rugby,
Warwickshire CV21 3AQ.
Tel. Rugby (0788) 61536

Crossroads (Scotland) Care Attendant Scheme: 24 George Square,
Glasgow G21 A9.
Tel. Glasgow (041) 226 3793

Distressed Gentle Folks Aid Association: Vicarage Gate House, Vicarage Gate,
London W8 4AQ.
Tel. 01 229 9341

Appendix 1

Help the Aged: 32 Dover Street, London W1A 2AP.
Tel. 01 499 0972

Jewish Welfare Board: 315/317 Ballards Lane, London N12 8LP.
Tel. 01 446 1499

The Marie Curie Foundation: 124 Sloane Street, London SW1X 9RF.

Methodist Homes for the Aged: 11 Tufton Street, London SW1P 3QD.
Tel. 01 222 0511

National Council for Voluntary Organizations: 26 Bedford Square, London WC1.
Tel. 01 636 4066

National Federation of Housing Associations: 30/32 Southampton Street, The Strand, London WC2E 7HE.
Tel. 01 240 2771/7

National Federation of Old Age Pensions Associations: (Pensioners' Voice): Melling House, 91 Preston New Road, Blackburn, Lancs B2 6BD.
Tel. Blackburn (0254) 52606

Pre-Retirement Association of Great Britain and Northern Ireland: 19 Undine Street, Tooting, London SW17 8PP.
Tel. 01 767 3225

Presbyterian Residential Trust: Church House, Fisherwick Place, Belfast BT1 6DW.
Tel. Belfast (0232) 22284

Retired Executives Action Clearing House (REACH): 1st Floor, Victoria House, Southampton Row, London WC1B 4DH.
Tel. 01 404 0940

Retirement Association of Northern Ireland: 42 Botanic Avenue, Belfast BT7 1JQ.
Tel. Belfast (0232) 21324

Royal British Legion: 49 Pall Mall, London SW1W 5JY.
Tel. 01 834 9353

Royal British Legion Scotland: New Haig House, Logie Green Road, Edinburgh EH7 4HR.
Tel. Edinburgh (031) 557 2782

Royal British Legion Wales: Area Organizer, 23 St. Andrews Crescent, Cardiff CF1 3QZ.
Tel. Cardiff (0222) 30216

Royal British Legion Northern Ireland: War Memorial Building, 9–13 Waring Street, Belfast BT12 DW.
Tel. Belfast (0232) 29988

Salvation Army: (HQ) 101 Queen Victoria Street, London EC4 4EP.
Tel. 01 236 7020

Scottish Federation of Housing Associations: 42 York Place, Edinburgh
EH1 3HU.
Tel. Edinburgh (031) 556 1435

Scottish Old Age Pensions Association: 12 Gordon Street, Lochgelly, Fife
PY5 9PT.
Tel. Lochgelly (0592) 780122

Task Force: (HQ) 1 Thorpe Close, London W10 5XL.
Tel. 01 960 5666

Women's Royal Voluntary Service: 17 Old Park Lane, London W1Y 4AJ.
Tel. 01 499 6040

Appendix 2. The coroner

To a certain extent coroners themselves determine what information they require after a death has occurred, if any is necessary at all. The coroner's officer, usually a police officer especially seconded to work with the coroner, is always pleased to inform doctors of the local coroner's views and statutory requirements. The coroner's officer is also usually very experienced and able to give unofficial as well as official advice about the best way of approaching a particular problem, and will always advise when there is any doubt about the need to refer a particular case. In general, however, if there is indeed any doubt it is better to refer the matter to the coroner. Referral is usually necessary if a death occurs without any obvious cause within 24 hours of admission to hospital, and this is so even when it is the local community or cottage hospital that is involved. Any suggestion of 'unnatural means' having contributed to a patient's demise also necessitates automatic referral to the coroner. Finally, any situation in which the issue of a death certificate presents difficulties, especially if there is a possibility of violence, should also automatically be discussed with the coroner.

The coroner and the coroner's officer are usually extremely helpful, making it their responsibility to look after the proper interests of the medical profession, as well as members of the general public. An inquest rarely results following the referral of a death to the coroner unless the circumstances are exceptional, although a post mortem will often be necessary.

Appendix 3. Compulsory institutionalization

COMPULSORY HOSPITALIZATION OF PSYCHIATRICALLY ILL PATIENTS

This is occasionally necessary in the elderly both in the case of the ambulant or aggressive demented patient and in those older people suffering with other psychiatric conditions. One or other of the sections of the 1959 Mental Health Act is most commonly invoked.

(i) Section 25 – admission for observation. Admission under Section 25 allows compulsory detention for up to 28 days. It can be prolonged while the patient is in hospital by application for admission for treatment under Section 26, which is discussed below. The requirements for Section 25 are:

An application for admission to hospital by the patient's nearest relative, or a person to whom the nearest relative had delegated authority (in this situation a copy of the authority is required), or a social worker who has had, if possible, prior consultation with the nearest relative.

Medical recommendation by two doctors who declare that the patient is suffering from mental disorder necessitating hospital detention, and that detention is necessary in the interest of his own health or safety, or for the protection of others, and that an informal admission is inappropriate.

The regulations state that one of the doctors should be approved by the Area Health Authority as being suitable to take action in these matters by virtue of his special experience, and the other should, wherever possible, have known the patient previously. This is usually the general practitioner's role. Both medical practitioners must sign the medical recommendations on or before the date of the application and they must examine the patient together, or within seven days of each other. The doctors and the applicant must also have seen the patient within fourteen days of the application having been made, and the patient must be admitted within fourteen days of the application being lodged.

There are also other regulations of a complex nature concerning the relationship between the applicant, the patient and the doctors. These will be known to the doctor who has been approved by the Area Health Authority to act under Section 25 and will not be detailed here.

(ii) Section 26 – admission for treatment. This allows detention of a patient for up to one year. The regulations are altogether of a more complex nature and it is less commonly invoked in the psychogeriatric situation. It is unlikely to involve the general practitioner and it is best left to the approved psychiatrist.

(iii) Section 29 – admission for observation in an emergency. This Section is appropriate for a patient suffering with mental disorder of a sufficient severity to require hospital detention if informal admission is inappropriate. It is also inherent in this Section that other measures to deal with the emergency would lead to inordinate delay. Initially, detention for 72 hours is allowed, but this can be extended for another 28 days. It requires:

An application for admission by a relative or social worker.

A medical recommendation, if possible from a doctor who has previously known the patient, which must be signed on or before the date of application.

That the patient has been seen by the applicant within three days of the application being made, and that the patient be admitted to hospital within three days of examination on the basis of which the medical recommendation has been made.

As described for Section 25, the relationship between the applicant, the patient and the doctor is governed by special regulations which will be known to the approved psychiatrist.

Appendix 4. A table of normal values in the elderly

Serum/plasma	SI units
Albumin	33–50 g/l
Alkaline phosphatase	2–14 KA units per 100 ml
Bilirubin – men	2–17 μmol/l
– women	3–12 μmol/l
Calcium	2.2–2.6 mmol/l
	(possibly as high as 2.85 mmol/l in women)
Creatinine	52–160 μmol/l
ESR – men	0–20 mm but see text
– women	0–30 mm
Glucose (random)	3.5–9.3 mmol/l
Haemoglobin	14.g/dl
LDH	100–530 units/ml
Potassium	3.5–5.5 mmol/l
SGOT (aspartate transaminase)	10–40 units/ml
Sodium	135–145 mmol/l
T4	58–128 nmol/l
T3	1.5–3.00 nmol/l
TSH	0–6 mu/l
Urea	4–10 mmol/l

References

Arie, T. (1981). *Health needs of the elderly.* Croom Helm, London. Other stimulating collections of essays are *Care of the elderly,* edited by A. N. Exton-Smith and J. Grimley Evans (Academic Press, London, 1977), and *The Impact of Ageing,* edited by David Hobman (Croom Helm, London, 1981).
Asher, R. (1974). The dangers of going to bed. *B. med. J.* ii, 967–8.
Balint, M. (1970). *Treatment or diagnosis. A study of repeat prescribing in general practices.* Tavistock, London.
Baxendale, C. *et al.* (1978). A self-medication retraining programme. *B. med. J.* ii, 1278–9.
Becker, M. H. (1974). *The health belief model and personal health behaviour.* Charles B. Slack, London.
Blaxter, M. (1976). *The meaning of disability.* Heinneman, London. In addition see the *Survey of handicapped and impaired in Great Britain,* HMSO, London, 1971, conducted by Amelia Harris for the Office of Population Censuses and Surveys. It is a mine of useful data on disability and handicap.
Bluebond-Lancer, M. (1978). *The private worlds of dying children.* Princeton University Press.
Blythe, R. (1979). *The view in winter reflections of old age.* Allen Lane, London.
Brearley, P. (1975). *Social work ageing and society.* Routledge and Kegan Paul, London.
—— (1978). *The social challenge of ageing* (ed. D. Hobman). Age and Social Work. Croom Helm, London.
British Medical Journal (1977). Deafness and mental health. *Br. med. J.* i, 191.
Brockington, C. F. and Lempert, S. M. (1966). *The social needs of the over 80s.* Manchester University Press.
Cartwright, A. and Anderson, R. (1981). *General practice revisited. A second study of patient and their doctors.* Tavistock, London.
—— Hockey, L., and Anderson, J. (1973). *Life before death.* Routledge and Kegan Paul, London.
Chapman, J. A. and Goodall, J. (1980). Helping a child to live whilst dying. *Lancet* i, 753.
Cullinan, T. R. (1978). Visually disabled people at home. *Hlth Trends* 10, 90–2.
Department of Health and Social Security (1972). A nutritional survey of the elderly at home. Report on Health and Social Subjects No. 3, London.
—— (1978). A happier old age. A discussion document on elderly people in our Society, London.
—— (1980). A nutritional survey of the elderly at home. Report on Health and Social Subjects No. 16. London.
Department of Health and Social Security, Scottish Office, Welsh Office, Northern Ireland Office (1981). Growing older. Command 8173. HMSO, London.
Disabled Living Foundation (1979). *The elderly person with failing vision.*
Drury, M. (1981). *The medical secretary's handbook,* 4th ed. Baillière, London.
Fentem, P. H. and Bassey, J. (1978). *The case for exercise.* Sports Council. This is an excellent brief summary of the benefits of exercise with all the main references added, giving a much more detailed and therefore much larger account of the subject is *Physical activity and ageing* by R. J. Shephard (Croom Helm, London, 1981).

Fox, R. H., Woodward, P. M., Exton-Smith, A. N., Green, M. F., Donnison, D. V., and Wicks, M. H. (1973). *Br. med. J.* i, 200–6. The full report of this study is *Old and cold* by Malcolm Wicks (Heinemann, London, 1978). In addition *The elderly at home* by Audrey Hunt (HMSO, London, 1978) gives very useful information about the types of heating used by elderly people.

Gilkes, M. J. (1979). Eyes run on light. *Br. med. J.* i, 1681–3.

Grad, J. and Sainsbury, P. (1965). An evaluation of the effects of caring for the aged at home. In *Psychiatric disorders in the aged*. Geigy.

Gray, J. A. M. (1980). Section 47: an ethical dilemma for doctors. *Hlth Trends* 3, 72–4.

—— and Mackenzie, M. (1979). *Take care of your elderly relative*. Allen Unwin/Beaconsfield. This is a relatives handbook summarizing all the main benefits and services available for relatives who are caring for an elderly parent.

—— and Wilcock, G. K. (1981). *Our elders*. Oxford University Press.

Hannay, D. R. (1979). *The symptom iceberg. A study of community health*. Routledge and Kegan Paul, London.

Hart, J. Tudor (1980). *Hypertension*. Churchill-Livingstone, Edinburgh.

Herbst, K. G. and Humphrey, C. (1980). Hearing impairment and mental state in the elderly living at home. *Br. med. J.* ii, 903–5.

Hinton, J. (1972). *Dying*. Penguin, Harmondsworth.

Hunt, A. (1978). *The elderly at home*. HMSO, London.

Isaacs, N. (1971). Geriatric patients: do their families care? *Br. med. J.* iii, 282–6.

Jolley, D. (1981). Dementia, misfits in need of care. In *Health care of the elderly* (ed. T. Arie) pp. 71–88. Croom Helm, London.

Kastenbaum, R. and Aisenberg, R. (1974). *The psychology of death*. Duckworth, London.

Knox, J. D. E. (1980). Prescribing for the elderly in general practice. A review of current literature. *J. R. Coll. Gen. Pract.* 30, Suppl. 1. See also the article Improving compliance – general practice, by J. M. Graham and D. A. Supree, in *J. R. Coll. Gen. Pract.* 29, 399–404 (1979).

Kubler-Ross, E. (1969). *On death and dying*. Macmillan, New York.

Miall, W. E. and Chinn, S. (1973). Blood pressure and ageing: results of a 15–17 year follow-up study in South Wales. *Clin. Sci. molec. Med.* 45, 238.

Moroney, R. M. (1976). *The Family and the State*. Longman. This short book makes stimulating and encouraging reading, reviewing the friends in family care for elderly and mentally handicapped people.

Murdoch, J. C. (1980). The epidemiology of prescribing in an urban general practice. *J. R. Coll. Gen. Pract.* 30, 593–602.

Nordin, C. (1978). Osteoporosis and osteomalacia. *Medicine*, 3rd series, No. 10. 491–500.

Norman, A. (1977). *Transport and the elderly*. NCCOP.

Office of Health Economics (1979). *Dementia in old age*. London.

Parkes, C. M. (1975). *Bereavement*. Penguin, Harmondsworth.

—— (1978). Home or hospital. *J. R. Coll. Gen. Pract.* 28, 19–30.

Pritchard, P. M. M. (1981). *Manual of primary health care,* 2nd edn. Oxford University Press.

——, Low, K., and Whalen, M. (1982). *Management in general practice*. Oxford University Press.

Rowntree, B. S. (1947). *Report of a survey committee on the problems of ageing and the care of old people*. Nuffield Foundation.

Royal College of General Practitioners (1981*a*). *Health and prevention in primary care*. Report from General Practice No. 18. London.

—— (1981*b*). *Prevention of arterial disease in general practice*. Report from General Practice No. 19. London.

—— (1981*c*). *Patient participation in general practice*. Occasional Paper No. 17. London.

Rubin, I. *et al.* (1975). *Improving the coordination of care. A program for health team development.* Ballinger, Cambridge, Mass.
Russell, M. A. H. *et al.* (1979). Effect of general practitioners' advice against smoking. *Br. med. J.* **ii**, 231–5.
Sackett, D. L. and Haynes, R. B. (1976). *Compliance with therapeutic regimens.* Johns Hopkins.
Saltin, B., Blanquist, G., Mitchell, J. M., Johnson, R. L., Wildenthall, K., and Chapman, C. B. (1968). Response to exercise after bed rest and after training. *Circulation* **38**, Suppl. VII.
Saunders, C. (1978). *Management of terminal disease.* Arnold, London.
Shegog, R. F. A. (ed.) (1981). *The impending crisis of old age: a challenge to ingenuity. A report and essays.* Oxford University Press for Nuffield Provincial Hospitals Trust.
Sheldon, J. H. (1948). *The social medicine of old age.* Oxford.
Stott, N. and Davis, R. H. (1979). The exceptional potential in each primary care consultation. *Jnl. R. Coll. Gen. Pract.* **29**, 201–5.
Tulloch, A. J. (1981). Repeat prescribing for elderly patients. *Br. med. J.* **282**, 1647–54.
—— and Moore, V. (1979). A randomized controlled trial of geriatric screening and surveillance in general practice. *J. R. Coll. Gen. Pract.* **29**, 733–42. For a more detailed analysis of screening see Williamson, J. (1981) and the descriptions of practical approaches to screening see pages 91–115 in *The care of the elderly in the community* By Idris Williams (Croom Helm, London, 1979), and the paper on Assessment of the elderly – general practice by J. H. Barber and J. B. Wallis (1976), *J. R. Coll. Gen. Pract.* **26**, 106–14.
Twycross, R. and Ventafridda, V. (1980). *The continuing care of terminal cancer patients.* Pergamon, Oxford.
Williamson, J. (1981). Screening surveillance and case finding. In *Health care of the elderly* (ed. T. Arie), pp. 194–214. Croom Helm, London.
——, Stokoe, I. H., Gray, S., Fiser, M., Smith, A., McGhee, A., and Stephenson, E. (1964). Old people at home, their unreported needs. *Lancet* **i**, 1117–20.
Wolff, H. (1980). The use of technology in the care of the elderly and disabled. In *Tools for living* (ed. J. Bray and S. Wright). Commission of European Communities, London.
Wood, P. H. N. (1980). The language of disablement. *International Rehabilitation Medicine,* **2**, 86–92.

Index

accidents, prevention of 213–14
agoraphobia 198
age
  biological 14
  chronological 14
Age Concern 206
aging, theories of 15
ageism 120
alcohol abuse 134
alkaline phosphatase 59
Alzheimer's disease 28
anaemia 18
  macrocytic 19
  microcytic 18
  normochromic/normocytic 19
ankle oedema 65
antidepressants 98
antidiuretic hormone, inappropriate secretion of 44
antihypertensive therapy 96
antimicrobials 97
arterial disease
  prevention of 201
  and smoking 202
arthritis 20, 33
  osteoarthritis 20, 23, 33
  rheumatoid arthritis 20, 33
aspartate transaminase 60
ataxia, cerebellar 33

backache 22
bacteriuria, asymptomatic 75
Balint, M. 216
Baxendale, C. 217
beliefs of older people about disease 112–19
bereavement, counselling 227, 231
bilirubin 60
blindness, *see* visual impairment
blood pressure, levels of 203–4

Cartwright, A. 203, 205
cataract 83
cerebrovascular accident 23
  aetiology 24
  brain stem 25
  cortex 25
  internal capsule 24
cervical spondylosis 32
chiropody 46–7
community hospitals 104
community involvement 206

community psychiatric nurses 200
community services 200
compliance, drug taking 90
confusion 26
  acute confusional states 27
  and isolation 196
constipation in terminal illness 225

day care 108
day hospital 101
deafness 35–7
death, place and cause of 219
deep venous thrombosis 20
dementia 28, 200
dependence, definition of 8, 196
dental problems 64
diabetes mellitus 24
  amyotrophy 34
  drug therapy 97
digoxin 95
disability
  assessment of 156
  definition of 8, 11
  early detection 205–12
  equipment for 200
  financial benefits for 180
district nurse 206–8, 211, 215–16
diuretics 95
dizziness 80, 81
domiciliary visits 101
dressing, problems 164
Drury, M. 217
dysphagia 29

epidemiology
  of fractures 213
  of prescribing 217
epilepsy 33
erythrocyte sedimentation rate 29

falls 31, 213
  management 34
family problems 138–55
femur, fracture of 2, 213–14
fire, risk of 194
fitness 3, 6, 131–3
folic acid, deficiency of 19
foot problems 46

gastrointestinal tract
  malabsorption 62
  malignancy 86

general practice
  changes in   200
  prescribing in   216–17
  prevention in   201, 214
  team work in   214
general practitioner
  and accidents   213
  and prescribing   217
  and prevention   201, 205, 206–9
  and teamworking   214–16
  workload of   199
geriatric screening   205–12
giddiness   80, 81
glaucoma   82, 83
gout   22

handicap
  definition of   8
  management of   156–70
  prevalence of   2
Hannay, D.   206
Hart, J. Tudor   202–3, 214
Health Education Council   202, 213
health visitor   200, 206–7, 210, 213
hearing loss   35–7
heating problems   190–4
hemiplegia   215; see also cerebrovascular accident
home-help   104
hospital admission in terminal illness   229
housework, problems with   166
housing problems   182–8
  of relatives   154
humerus, fracture of   2
hypocalcaemia   37
  treatment   224
hyperglycaemia   38
  complications   39
  treatment   39
hypertension, detection and treatment of   202–5
hypnotics   92
hypoalbuminaemia   40
hypocalcaemia   41
hypokalaemia   42
hyponatraemia   44
hypotension, postural   31, 213
hypothermia   45, 206
  prevention of   190–4

intrinsic team   215
immobility   9, 45, 124
incontinence
  faecal   48
  urinary   50
    apparent   50
    counselling   198
    isolation and   198
    management   54

  nocturnal   55
  psychological   53
  retention with overflow   51
  stress   52
  uninhibited neurogenic bladder   53
  and vaginitis   52
insomnia, affecting relatives   153
isolation   124, 195

jaundice
  drugs and   58
  haemolytic   58
  hepatocellular   58
  obstructive   57

ketonuria   40
Knox, J.   217

lactic acidosis   40
lactic dehydrogenase   59
loneliness   195
longevity   15

malabsorption   62
malnutrition   62, 166
Miall, W. E.   202
mobility
  aids   48
  problems   9
morbidity, patterns of   7
Murdoch, J. C.   217
musculo-skeletal disorders   206
myocardial infarction   65
myopathy, proximal   34

National Assistance Act 1948   119
Nordin, C.   214
nursing the dying   226, 228
nutritional problems and isolation   196

occupational therapy   160
old people's homes   106, 187
orthopaedic services   105
osteomalacia   23, 67
osteoporosis   22, 68, 213

patient participation   206
Paget's disease   23, 38, 69
pain, treatment of in terminal illness   222–4
pancreas, carcinoma of   87
parkinsonism   33, 69
  therapy   96
peptic ulceration   87
pets, benefit of   198
physiotherapy   20, 21, 160
Plummer–Vinson syndrome   29
polymyalgia rheumatica   71
population changes
  age distribution   200
  number of elderly   220

poverty 126, 176–82
  of relatives 154
practice nurse 204–5, 216
pre-retirement education 129
prescribing 90–9, 209, 212, 216–18
pressure sores 71
prevention 127–37, 201–12, 214
  of accidents 213–14
  of family problems 145–8
Pritchard, P. M. M. 200, 215–16
proteinuria 74
pseudo-gout 22
psychiatric hospitals 106

relatives, problems of 138–55
relocation effect 109
renal failure 72
  acute 74
  chronic 73
repeat prescription cards 217
residential care 106, 187
retinopathy 83
Royal College of General Practitioners
  (RCGP) 201, 202, 206
Royal Society for Prevention of Accidents
  213
Rubin, I. 216
Russell, M. A. H. 243

Section 47 119
self-care problems 11
self-help groups 202, 206
self-medication 133
single daughters, problems of 155
sleep problems affecting relatives 152–3
smoking 201
  and arterial disease 202
social problems 171–98
social security 177
social services for elderly people 172–4
social workers 102, 172–6
Stott, N. 202

stroke 23; *see also* cerebrovascular accident
subdural haematoma 75
supporters of the elderly 200, 215–16

team work 214–16
telephones 124
temporal arteritis 24, 76
thyroid disorders 76
  hypothyroidism 76
  thyrotoxicosis 78
toe nails, cutting of 46
tranquillizers 94
transient ischaemic attacks 33
tuberculin test 79
tuberculosis 79
Tulloch, A. J. 205

ulcers
  ischaemic 61
  leg 61
  pressure sore 61
  stasis 61
  varicose 61
urobilinogen 60

vertigo 31, 80
visual impairment 87
  acute 82
  advice to relatives 85
  aids for 84
  chronic 83
  mental health and 84
vitamin B_{12} 19
voluntary organizations 168–71, 206
volunteers 168
vomiting, treatment of 224

washing and bathing problems 164
weight loss 86
  check-list 86
Wolff, H. 200

4) I just asked Doctor if he could go to hospital either
1. I don't want him to go
to Keswick or Attingham or else we shall
[illegible] to explain
I can manage except when he is v. confused & ill or an
attack – but apparently hospital staff wouldn't dare have him e.g. let me have done?
2. He is much better at home
(effect of Hospital & Audrey) [illegible]
  always [illegible] He hated hospital Keswick wouldn't want him ill like that.
3. Any [illegible] must be discussed
with him [illegible] his reaction. Doctor doesn't
agree but surely his acceptance essential?
4. [illegible] Doctor [illegible]
be left on his own day [illegible] day
[illegible] Keswick only [illegible]
5. [illegible]
  Week [illegible]
6. I would suspect just he would
very likely try to "escape" home
  if it gets more [illegible]
What then?
  War Park — No — Doctor [illegible]
that Keswick [illegible]
as Kay would keep [illegible]
Kay"   C.S.B.S.

½ How much?

C S B F Home   Hoxham
Would there be a trial
N on [illegible] to me — Not
frequent visits — extra [illegible] — [illegible]
                                    home